Praise for *Aging Joyfully*

There are many ways to age, if we are fortunate enough to do it at all. No way comes without challenges that can't be avoided. But how we meet them and go beyond coping to experiencing joy and appreciation for the development and opportunities aging can bring is optional. Dr. Carla Marie Manly provides clear directions and insights for a successful, satisfying journey that rings true. This book is a life-changer that gives new meaning to the term "self help."

—Dr. Thelma Reese, coauthor (with Dr. Barbara Fleisher) of *The New Senior Woman: Reinventing the Years beyond Mid-Life* and *The New Senior Man: Exploring New Horizons, New Opportunities*

Aging Joyfully is an uplifting, essential read for every woman facing aging issues. Dr. Carla Marie Manly demonstrates beautifully that we each have the power to choose a path of joy in the inevitable aging journey. Dr. Manly's compassionate guidance promotes this essential shift: Aging can be beautifully empowering; it can offer every woman a new lease on life when its gifts are honored with grace and dedication. In the pages of *Aging Joyfully*, Dr. Manly moves the reader away from worry, doubt, and fear and into the creation of a most powerful, joyful future.

—Orchid D. Johnson MS, PhD, LMFT, LPCC, and Board Certified PTSD Clinician

In *Aging Joyfully*, Dr. Carla Marie Manly projects aging holistically using grace, mindfulness, and humor. I am eager to share her wisdom with friends, colleagues, and nursing students to encourage approaching women's aging with understanding, compassion, and empathy.

—Kathleen Rockett, MSN, RN, professor at Sonoma State University, BSN program

Aging Joyfully is a much-needed, empowering read for women of all ages. Whether you're in your 30s, 70s, or somewhere in between, this book takes the reader on an adventure into the heart and soul of womanhood. Dr. Carla Marie Manly's genuine, open style invites the reader to understand and embrace all aspects of her life. She covers a vast array of vital topics with clarity and ease. *Aging Joyfully* is a must-read for every woman who wants to live with intention and joy.

—Joan Tabb, MA, author of *Building Blocks for the NEW Retirement*

Aging Joyfully offers the reader extraordinary insights for creating a joy-filled life. Although the journey of aging can be discomforting in many ways, Dr. Carla Marie Manly offers the reader comprehensive, reassuring wisdom. With a tone that is at once gentle and intelligent, Dr. Manly guides the reader step-by-step into the realm of aging with joy and grace.

—Walter Tom, MD, FACS

In the pages of *Aging Joyfully*, Dr. Carla Marie Manly guides readers into a full appreciation of the freedom to be found in the later years of life. With an honest, humorous approach, she illuminates the unexpected delights of aging while offering expert insights into navigating aging challenges.

—Erica Manfred, author of *I'm Old, So Why Aren't I Wise?: Snarky Senior in the Sunshine State*

The blend of intelligence and compassion in this beautiful book should help many women deal with the real issues in getting older. You will find guidance, understanding, and a positive but not unrealistic approach to aging. Dr. Manly is an excellent writer and has deep experience, both of which make this book stand out. You can trust it and be inspired to be your best self.

—Thomas Moore, author of *Care of the Soul and Ageless Soul*

AGING

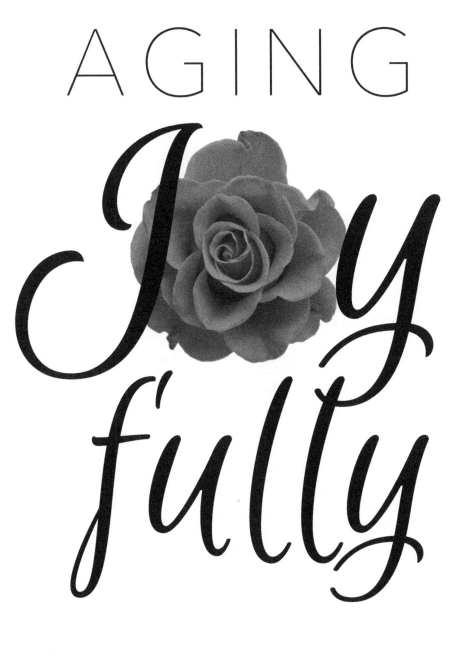

Joyfully

Published by Familius LLC, www.familius.com

Familius books are available at special discounts for bulk purchases, whether for sales promotions or for family or corporate use. For more information, contact Familius Sales at 559-876-2170 or email orders@familius.com.

Library of Congress Cataloging-in-Publication Data
2019935097

Print ISBN 9781641701419
Ebook ISBN 9781641702102

Printed in the United States of America

Edited by Laurie Duersch and Peg Sandkam
Cover design by Derek George and Carlos Guerrero
Book design by Brooke Jorden

10 9 8 7 6 5 4 3 2 1

First Edition

AGING

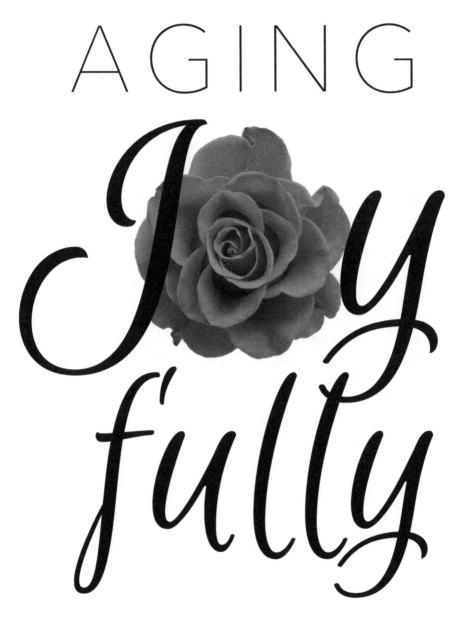

Joyfully

A Woman's Guide to Optimal Health,
Relationships, and Fulfillment for Her 50s and Beyond

CARLA MARIE MANLY, PHD

DEDICATION

This book is dedicated to you, the reader. Thank you for having the courage and desire to embrace the years before you with love and joy. *You* have the power to live every day of your life filled with purpose, passion, and delight. May you feel the light of my loving and supportive friendship throughout your journey.

Love, I am ever grateful to have you by my side and in my heart. Thank you for sharing this beautiful adventure of love and life with me. Love never fails.

Contents

Preface

It is one of my greatest privileges and joys in life to be a guide to others. My work has been informed by countless mentors, authors, and psychotherapists who have blessed me with their wisdom and talents. Many—from Carl Jung to Thomas Moore—have paved the way for me, and it is with humble gratitude that I honor their brilliant contributions to the world and my own life.

Given the poignant, intimate nature of this book and the aging process in general, it is important for the reader to consult with a primary care provider and engage professional psychological support whenever needed. As you journey into greater awareness and well-being, may you find and embrace the joy, love, and connection you so richly deserve.

Please note that the case studies and examples in this book are representative amalgamations. Although names and identifying details have been changed to protect privacy, the challenges and journeys are real. No story, case study, or example is intended to, nor do they, depict any singular person, event, or situation.

Introduction

*J*f you are a woman approaching—or already within—your fifties or sixties, it's likely that the array of changes you are encountering is at least somewhat disconcerting for you. From sagging skin and libido fluctuations to the uncharted territory of retirement, these changeable decades of life can be filled with oddities and unknowns. As a result, some women are absolutely terrified by the transition into their more mature years. Many feel an uneasy mixture of emotions, from occasional anxiety to chronic irritation. Some are angry as they fume in frustration at what seems like yet another stage in their forced march away from youth. Still others find joy and graceful ease in this new era of life, welcoming these interesting decades as a time to create greater individuality and freedom. These rare women seem to have discovered the art of aging with wisdom and powerful grace. If you find yourself yearning to join those who delight in these precious, mature years of life, *Aging Joyfully* is your warm and loving guide.

In truth, no book or doctor's waiting room can promise you a quick remedy for the challenges that might come your way. What I can offer you, however, is more valuable than any temporary cure. I can promise you this: When you embrace your journey with wisdom and loving awareness, you will find freedom through true understanding and acceptance. Your heart will be filled with joy and serenity as you come to appreciate and honor your life and the adventures ahead.

Within the pages of *Aging Joyfully*, you will be invited to discover and appreciate yourself as you transition into this next era of your life. You will be encouraged to embrace all that you are and become all that you have hoped to be. You will be encouraged to envision the woman you *want* to be. In looking at yourself and your world through the prism of personal choice—of how you *want* your life to unfold in these next decades—you will feel empowered. You will come to honor the wisdom, resilience, power, and grace you have already fostered in life. You will steadily come to use all that you have collected, and all that you are about to learn, to make your life more enjoyable and powerful. By taking a fresh and honest look at the path ahead—both the beckoning abundance and the bittersweet changes—you will find that fulfillment and joy await you in the days, months, and years ahead.

Your journey will also allow you to re-envision your conceptualization of the later decades of womanhood. During this process, you may come to focus more on the positive aspects of aging and all the gifts that greater maturity brings. In learning to honor your own maturing womanhood, you may come to embrace the power you have to influence your own life. As your understanding and awareness grow, you may find that you want your voice—your life—to be part of the shift that our youth-thirsty world sorely needs. Indeed, it is far too easy for maturing women to feel ashamed and alone in the aging process; it is time for this to change. If you desire to free yourself of the "youth-is-better" mindset (and the haunting, self-limiting fears that come with it), this is your opportunity. You, and only you, get to choose what, if anything, defines you as you age. This simple truth is one of the greatest benefits of being a mature woman: you are quite free to choose how you see and embrace this part of your journey.

These mature decades are unlike any other time in your life. Indeed, it is likely that you have no young children to tend to each day. Your career demands may have lessened. Your personal relationships may be more fine-tuned. You may have accomplished so many of the "musts" in life that you now can do as you choose. In many ways, you may have paid your dues by fulfilling endless obligations and now have time and space in your life to create and expand beyond your small or secret dreams. Your duty now is to yourself. Perhaps for the first time in your life, you can focus on that which brings you joy. This is your time to set your own standards, your own pace, and your own goals. Your later years bring you the gift of choice. This era of your life offers the opportunity to choose whatever allows you to age powerfully and joyfully—in ways that are uniquely and perfectly right for you.

I am mindful that these later decades of life are poignant ones. With all their promise of freedom and breathtaking transitions, a sense of loss can arise as we move from one phase of life to another. It would be disingenuous to pretend that this isn't so. The reality of life is that we are moving toward letting go from the moment we are born. The longer we journey through life, the more we find ourselves faced with fewer new beginnings and more natural endings. This is precious, hard truth; this is life. Yet life also tells us that new beginnings are always possible and that these later decades may allow us to cherish them more deeply.

Chronological time insists that you are getting older. And, indeed, your body may surely show signs of having served you well. Yet there is a precious treasure that is beyond the bodily changes and chronological time. This treasure is the indomitable spirit of the wild, graceful girl of your dreams. This childlike, fearless spirit knows no sense of time. This irrepressible spirit may have been cast aside or diminished during the earlier decades of your life, but she has been waiting for you all along. As you honor your eternally radiant spirit and meld it with the wisdom of your years, you will find the gifts and the true beauty of aging joyfully. You will discover that this time of your life is not a time to be feared, but another wondrous segment of self-art in progress.

In the pages of *Aging Joyfully*, we will journey together into the highs and lows of many sensitive, personal issues. We will explore the changes of the maturing body. We will delve into the process of reconciling with the self and moving forward without regret. We will investigate the dynamics of shifting relationships. We will honor the cycle of life that demands that we love and release all which we have loved so dearly. We will embrace all of this—and so much more—with conscious awareness, honesty, and positivity.

Aging does not need to be feared or faced alone. This is the beauty, the wonder, of being a woman. We can band together in love and community as only women can do. We can relish our commonalities and respect our precious differences. We can honor and support each other's choices, for powerful, graceful aging has no overarching plan. There is no one "right" way to age; there is only the way that is right for you—the way that honors you. As women who pause to honor each other at various stages in life (counting no stage as better or worse than another), we come to honor life itself. In this process, we not only foster love and respect for ourselves and each other, but for women of all ages who look to us for guidance—for learning how to be.

With a nod to the men in our lives, it is important to remember that they, too, often have substantial age-related fears. Although they may not suffer in the ways that women do, men also feel the bite of aging. Perhaps they are less conscious of and vocal about the changes and challenges of the aging process, yet men often possess some of the same fears. This often unspoken truth is important, for it can inform and guide you as you venture into the journey ahead. As we increase our self-awareness and knowledge as women, our compassionate wisdom can be channeled to create the changes we need and desire.

And so, I offer this book as a guide to embracing yourself as you may never have done in the past. This moment gives us the opportunity to be present and also glance into the future with hope and passion. *Let us work together to never lose sight of the beauty of aging.* Let us hold true, as partners, to the ideal of embracing this beautiful phase of life with vibrant, heartfelt gratitude.

Thank you for choosing to share your journey with me. I am blessed to age powerfully and joyfully with you.

With love and joy,
Carla Marie Manly

CHAPTER 1

Embracing Maturity with Wisdom and Joy

Your Beautiful Personal Journey

Welcome to one of the most beautiful eras of your life. This is a truly precious time and space, one in which you can come to honor your life, your aging process, and the gifts of your journey. If you're shaking your head in disbelief as you wonder how this could be one of the most beautiful times of your life, you've found the guidebook that is essential for you. Indeed, if you are willing to move through these pages with an open heart and mind, you will come to explore and know the inimitable depths and potential of your beautiful self.

Given that you are about to embark on a journey that will invite you to explore your inner and outer worlds, you might find it very helpful—even necessary—to have a journal specifically dedicated to this process. Choose your journal or notebook carefully, for it will ultimately hold some of your most sacred thoughts, emotions, dreams, and plans. This private journal will be a witness to your journey. Keep your journal and a writing implement by your side as you read this book. You may be drawn to make notes and complete exercises in the pages of your journal. As you progress, you will encounter a variety of "Wisdom Tips" (some of which contain exercises). Some may seem compelling and inviting while others may not. Feel free to customize tips and exercises to suit your personal needs. For example, certain exercises involve writing letters to yourself. If this sounds inviting, write to your heart's content; if not, feel free to make informal notes as thoughts, feelings, and images arise. Work in whatever ways feel right to you, allowing yourself the gift of consistent nonjudgment as to grammar, content, and form. Whatever you write or sketch is part of your unique process.

Note, too, that your process may surely be affected by the space in which you read this book. When possible, strive to read when you are feeling relaxed and undistracted by the outside world. Your mind and spirit will absorb your process more fully when you are able to be present to whatever thoughts and feelings arise. You will find that it is helpful to be in a tranquil, comfortable environment when you are reading and journaling. Always proceed when you feel both physically and psychologically ready.

Given the intimate, focused nature of this journey, it's important to respect your unique needs as to pacing and depth of work. If you feel that the timing or nature of an exercise is not appropriate for you, simply skip the exercise without judgment. As this book is not intended to be a replacement for necessary medical or psychological assistance, remember to reach out for professional support if the need arises. Indeed, overall self-awareness and self-care are vital elements of your overall journey.

The beauty of this journey rests in one simple truth: this is *your* process. The pace, depth, and nature of your unfolding are entirely up to you. It is your personal intention, willingness, and energy that will allow you to uncover and embrace the lasting joy and beauty that waits inside of you. There is no quick-fix for life's challenges; loving awareness and cultivated wisdom are your keys.

Age-Negative and Age-Positive Attitudes

If you are like me and the countless women I have talked with as a clinical psychologist, mentor, and friend, the idea of aging sometimes feels unpleasant on many levels. We live in a society where youth is coveted and older age is undesirable, unwanted, and even pathologized. Ageism (stereotyping and discriminating against an individual based upon age) can be tremendously offensive and challenging when encountered in the world at large. I am truly concerned that many women suffer from ageism perpetuated by others, as well as by what I have come to term "self-ageism." It is particularly sad, however, that many women consciously and unconsciously hold stereotypical attitudes and engage in negatively biased behaviors that are reflective of self-ageism. This is a powerful concept, for it can inspire energy for self-reflection and change.

It's easy to become caught in the unconscious reinforcement of ageism. A simple, yet significant shift is this: Youth does not equate to beauty. Beauty does not equate to youth. Yes, there is a certain beauty in youth, but we must not forget that there is also substantial, certain beauty in age. The two are, rightly, independent of each other, yet we slip into the space of wanting to compare and contrast the two. Age need never be in competition with youth; each has its own space.

Sadly, even women in their mid-twenties and early thirties have confided that they are fearful of getting old—of already *being* old—and worried that life is passing them by. So fearful have we become of the natural processes of aging that we are often terrified of natural lines, changing skin, and graying hair. With forty-year-olds sharing surreal tales of being carefully ousted at work in favor of younger, "smarter" brains, and thirty-somethings telling me that they are fearful of being winnowed out to make room for Generation Z, it is easy to see that something is amiss. Age has become something to fear, a wicked old witch to be avoided. Advertisers tell us we must fight this terrible foe at all costs. Youth-oriented ad campaigns promote age-targeted products and de rigueur cosmetic procedures that many women can ill afford. Yet countless women (some barely into their twenties) line up for the next product that promises youthful beauty.

You may be nodding in agreement and wondering what has become of our world—a world where women have become terrified of the aging process. It is tremendously unfortunate that our society has promoted an attitude that makes it nearly impossible for the everyday woman to believe it is possible to age with authenticity, power, and grace. Through what I have come to term as "age-negative attitudes," many women and men have consciously and unconsciously conspired to create the attitude that the aging process is a penalty—a dark abyss—that results in a woman eventually becoming undesirable, irrelevant, burdensome, and unwanted. Such attitudes take hold and often result in a woman actually believing that such "facts" are true.

Age-negative attitudes can have deep and far-reaching implications, for they hit at the very heart of an individual's core need to feel loved and safe. Age-positive attitudes, those that embrace aging as a naturally beautiful aspect of life, move away from the polarizing voice that says, "Youth is more desirable and valuable than older age." Age-positive attitudes embrace the truth that all stages in life offer both challenging and tremendously wonderful elements. When one stage or era is thought to be superior to another, the gifts of the other life stages can be minimized, devalued, and disregarded. Aging is not a negative process; it is a positive, incredibly rewarding part of life as a whole.

One particular client, who I will refer to as Marina, offers a compelling example of the often-hidden nature of aging issues.

Just shy of sixty, Marina is a stunning figure of womanhood in her curvaceous, au natural way. Artful lines grace the corners of her eyes, and the gentle creases near her lips evidence years of love and laughter. Marina wears no makeup and has allowed her thick, auburn hair to show its radiant strands of gray. With self-assured posture, a carefree attitude, and a firm sense of her business prowess, Marina seems to embody womanhood within (or possibly approaching) its prime. Yet the charming, self-assured exterior hides a host of secret fears. Inside, like many maturing women, Marina is terrified.

Her private, fearful woes include concerns of a waning libido, changing appearance, and age discrimination. Marina confided her secret fear that her loving, faithful husband will one day wake up and find her unattractive. She holds deep worries for her parents and her financial security. In one session, Marina's composed exterior cracked as she began to cry.

"I am so worried," she said, "that I will lose my health. I am terrified that some terrible disease—Alzheimer's or cancer—will take over my life. I am worried that I'll decline and lose my independence. I never want to be a burden to anyone. I want to live long and well, fully capable of caring for myself and my loved ones."

It wasn't Marina's changing appearance and shifting libido that worried her most; it was what these changes represented—her fear of losing the resilience, strength, and suppleness of her youth. She feared the loss of her dearly prized personal power and independence. On a foundational level, Marina's fears told of her very normal need to feel valuable, loved, and safe. Some of Marina's fears were valid and needed attention. Yet most of her fears were self-torturing demons with no basis in truth. All of them shared one characteristic: they conspired and worked together to keep Marina from embracing and enjoying her current life as fully as possible.

Marina's story reveals many of the common fears that haunt women as they move forward in life. From women in their early thirties to those in their mid-seventies, many have offered stories that share various age-related themes with Marina's. Although an age-negative script is more common from those in their mid-forties onward, the reality is that many women fear aging from a fairly early age.

Although it certainly may be more pronounced and widespread in today's world, the anti-aging trend isn't new. Women have long feared being cast aside for their younger counterparts. History is filled with tales of searches for youth-inducing elixirs and anti-aging potions, yet certain cultures and bygone eras also knew the importance of honoring older women for their gifts of wisdom, dignity, and timeless beauty. When this attitude is present, when age and maturity are embraced for their gifts and virtues, a reverence for all stages of womanhood results. Without this lack of appreciation and awareness, the more mature, luminous years of a woman's life can be sadly devalued. Such mindsets not only promote the disrespect of decades of womanhood, they also promote the waste of vast wisdom and power. In truth, age-negative attitudes foster the waste of empowering energy and of life itself.

Many women feel tempted—or even forced—to lie about their age. This is ageism at work in a most pernicious form. I cringe when I hear stories of women who have been advised to lie about their age on job applications, shave off a few years or more when creating an online dating profile, or have felt it necessary to downsize their age in social settings.

I received a newsletter recently that made my heart sink. The author noted that she'd been advised by an executive recruiter to "shave ten years off" of her experience, or in other words, her age. The newsletter also noted that women age fifty or older "may need to lie" about age and experience when looking for a new job. Knowing that the author is a women's advocate, I read the newsletter several times in disbelief.

Many women tell me that they've been compelled to alter their age when dating. As one client told me, "Everyone does it—both men and women. If I don't lie about my age, then I'm automatically out of my league. When other sixty-year-olds are claiming they are in their fifties, then men are drawn to them, not me. But it's not only women. The men on the site who are matched to me say they are in their sixties, but I'm finding that quite a few are in their seventies. It feels like a game." Dishonesty ultimately hurts everyone.

Although, historically, many women have felt compelled to state their age as lower than their actual years, there is no reason for this trend to continue. In fact, there is every reason for women to be proud of their age; it's just a number. A woman's age does not reflect who she is; a number sheds no light on a woman's capacities, intelligence, spirit, soul, and overall being. Personally, I refuse to take part in any practice or movement that suggests that I lie about my age or any aspect of my being. If we do not take a stand against foundational issues such as this, then we are part of the problem of perpetuating ageism. It's time that we take a stand for truth and honesty. It's time that we, as women, refuse to engage in behaviors that are ultimately harmful to the ideal of aging with pride, joy, and grace.

Let's face it head-on. It's time that we upend the mindset that aging is negative and that youth is inherently superior. In fact, it's well past the time that we allow ourselves to be diminished—rather than heralded—for the magnificent gifts we have accrued through the journey of life. Rather than "fighting" the aging process, wouldn't it be lovely to own it, embrace it, and make it our own? This is achievable. Through making wise, tailor-made personal choices that allow you to be the best, most brilliant version of yourself at any age, you can be gorgeous from the inside out at *every* age.

This doesn't mean that you'll be free of issues related to aging. However, it does mean that you will feel empowered and free as you face what comes your way. It means, too, that you will become a woman who proudly embraces and models her mature womanhood. You will become a poster child—a poster *woman*—for the wise, beautifully radiant power that can come with a woman's later years. If you find yourself smiling at the thought or even wondering if I'm offering you a dream, I understand. Shake off any doubt, for your soul knows the truth: You are far more than any number or projected image; you cannot be defined by your chronological age. You are more than the sum of your years on this planet. You are a woman who is filled with the power of resilience, wisdom, and vast life experience.

The Power of Mindset Maneuvers

As you begin your journey into the art of powerful and joyful aging, remember that your mindset is what matters most. You are affected by your inner dialogue far more than you might know. If the tape running inside your head is negative and critical, you will likely view the world in a negative, judgmental way. Any disparaging thoughts you have ultimately translate into unhelpful words and behaviors. In the same way, a positive mindset will translate into a view of the world that is largely optimistic and nonjudgmental. The uplifting, kind thoughts you hold inside will be translated into positive words and actions. These concepts are age-old truths and are reflected in phrases such as "pretty is as pretty does" and John Milton's, "The mind is its own place, and in itself / Can make a Heav'n of Hell, a Hell of Heav'n" (*Paradise Lost*, 1667). The power of one's mindset cannot be denied.

If you engage in self-ageism and look at your aging process as a dark and gloomy march away from youth and toward decrepitude, then your mindset may likely make it so. If, instead, you choose to look at this time in your life as though you are on the verge of a most (if not *the* most) spectacular phase of your life, then it will be so. Your mind has this incredible power within it. You can choose to make a heaven—not a hell—out of this era of your life. Your mindset is truly *everything* in shaping your ability to age joyfully.

During a recent visit, a dear friend shared her journey into aging with me. Captivated by her witty insights, I listened with empathy and delight.

With bright, laughing eyes she noted, "I used to think I had to wait until later in life to be happy. I thought that happiness would be something I would 'get to' eventually. I muddled through the first six decades of my life thinking I would find happiness if I did this or that or after I changed this or that. The not-so-silent tape in my mind said, 'Everything has to be "thus and so" and *then* I will be happy.' Now, at this stage in my life, I've realized that true happiness doesn't need to be 'found.' It's right here in front of me if I just stop to enjoy it. But that's one of the beauties of being in my golden years; I'm less flustered and pressured. My attitude is far different. I don't resist life. I don't resist aging. I don't chase happiness. I see the beauty in every day."

As the conversation took a more retrospective turn, she shared intimate details of her distant past. Although the subject matter was laden with tales of hardships and hurts, her attitude was one of wise acceptance.

"You know," she said with a gentle softness that was matched by the warmth in her eyes, "I don't ache about my past as I once did. I don't mourn the loss of that time in my life—what I often referred to as my 'wasted years.' I've come to see that period as necessary for my growth. I couldn't see it at the time, but in hindsight I have come to realize that I ultimately learned and grew into the woman I am now."

She laughed brightly and said, "It certainly took a lot of time for me to absorb certain lessons, but I'm hardheaded that way. I needed to learn in my own time. And when I was ready, I certainly did learn and move forward. I used to beat myself up about my past and the time I thought I wasted, but now I embrace all of it. It's part of who I am and certainly nothing to lament or be ashamed of in any way. There's no use in expending any energy ruminating on the past. I've learned from my experiences, and I used them to become a better woman—a woman I am increasingly proud to be. More than ever, I am getting out of my comfort zone to explore *new* parts of myself. Learning and growing—isn't that what matters most?"

I smiled at my dear, wise friend. She radiated with a peaceful luminosity. By changing her mindset from one of fear and negativity to one of joy and positivity, she found a key secret to aging with power and grace.

Of course, such attitudes are often hard won. Depending upon your unique personality and history, it can be difficult to live in positivity. Some people seem to be born optimists, whereas others seem to naturally view life through a lens of pessimism. Of course, even generally positive individuals can become circumspect and jaded as a result of difficult personal experiences. Our later years allow us the opportunity to pause, re-evaluate our attitudes, and move forward in ways that give us greater joy and ease.

Taylor, a strong-willed woman in her early sixties, sought my assistance in moving out of what she termed an "aging funk." Taylor listed her complaints with life in a dry, brittle voice:

"I don't know what's happened to me. I used to be an upbeat person, the go-to girl, but I've become a drab, worn-out version of who I used to be. Even my marriage has become dull and routine. It's the same every day; we go to work, come home, watch television, and then go to bed. Sex is a thing of the past; neither of us seem to have any interest. We used to have fun on the weekends, and we used to travel every chance we got. But after my husband's heart surgery, we rarely do anything outside our dreary routine. In the past, we would ride our bikes and go for long hikes together, but now it's a big deal to take the dog for a five-minute walk.

"My father-in-law, who used to be a pillar of health, has cancer and is failing rapidly; his suffering really weighs on us. I wish I had a cure, but I don't. It might sound selfish, but it's such a downer to go see him in the nursing home. In the past, I would have had a far different attitude, but something's shifted in me. Even my friendships seem stagnant; I'm tired of the same unproductive chatter and stories.

"My job, which once meant everything to me, is going nowhere but downhill. I used to be so passionate about my work. I was the best at what I did, but that's not the case any longer. Even the work atmosphere has changed. With so many youngsters in the ranks, I feel outdated. I am past my prime. I know it, and others know it too. I never thought I'd say this, but the younger staff members are smarter than me. They do their jobs better. I am just too old. I can feel it every day. It's all about survival of the fittest, and they are smarter and fitter than me. I tell you, it's a dark, competitive world out there."

Indeed, Taylor had sunk into an age-related period of depression. One might say that Taylor was trapped in self-ageism. Her grim, negative outlook mirrored her darkening interior world. Faced with challenging issues, such as her husband's heart surgery and father-in-law's decline, Taylor had unwittingly slipped into a state of depression. Accustomed to being in control of her world, it was difficult for Taylor to adjust to the truth that many of the challenges she was facing were beyond her control. As a result, unconscious feelings of helplessness and frustration added to her angst.

Her mental and emotional unrest was worsened by the change in her exercise patterns and daily routines. Taylor's lifestyle had shifted from being active and adventurous to sedate and routine. Her work identity, too, had shifted. Proud of always being "the best" at her job, she no longer felt valuable and "on top of her game." Taylor's sense of power and positivity had diminished as all of these issues (and more) moved in and festered inside of her. Over time, Taylor's fears, hurts, and complaints overshadowed her naturally upbeat nature. Taylor's goal, then, was to face her issues, address what she could with positivity, and release herself from the negative weight of all that was beyond her control.

Of course, many serious mental health issues (e.g., major depressive disorder) require far more than a "shift in attitude." Serious mental health concerns require professional attention that often includes psychotherapy and appropriate psychopharmacological medications. Although depression and other mental health concerns will be addressed more fully in chapter 2, it's important to emphasize that such issues need and deserve proper attention.

There is great wisdom in seeking professional assistance when life seems too heavy or difficult to manage alone. Outside assistance, whether from your physician, psychotherapist, or skilled mentor, can provide beneficial guidance and tools to support your journey.

But with or without such challenges, you can come to feel truly empowered knowing this phase in your life comes with the great opportunity to redefine yourself—your attitudes, your behaviors, and your way of being in the world. An age-positive attitude will be one of your greatest resources in your journey. So wherever you lie on the spectrum of positivity (be it at the especially optimistic pole, downright pessimistic pole, or somewhere in between), know that your attitude does make a difference. Although you might not be able to quickly shift your outlook a complete 180-degrees, trust that you can take steps toward embracing an attitude that gives you greater joy and ease.

Now is the time to begin noticing if self-ageism (or any form of ageism) is negatively impacting your life. Now is the time to notice, embrace, and feed your positive inner power. The nature of your attitude has a great impact during all phases of your life, yet the quality of your later years can be particularly affected by your outlook. Isn't it absolutely amazing that you—beautiful you—have such power inside yourself?

Your Subjective Age

Several years ago, I attended a lecture offered by an extraordinary woman who had guided me in many ways. Although I had never met her in person, I'd read her books, learned from her wisdom, and patterned aspects of my life upon her teachings. It wasn't until she was in her early eighties that I finally met her, and I was captivated by her radiant beauty.

Perhaps her face was lined and creased with years of love-filled living. Perhaps her hair was gray and wispy. Perhaps her body—the home to her beautiful heart—was thin and fragile. Yet it was not any superficial qualities that held my attention. What I did notice and absorb was this woman's light. She possessed a rare, luminous quality that made the thought of chronological years a nonissue. The moment she took my hand and gazed into my eyes—when her soul touched mine for an instant—I saw deep, eternal beauty. This wise, incredible woman was ageless. In that moment, I felt the power she held—the power she had earned—through her conscious, inspiring journey in life. Her unforgettable, shimmering eyes possessed the sparkle of a child's wonder, the compassion of a mother's love, and the knowing brilliance of a revered elder's wisdom. That brief intersection of our worlds changed me. Without my knowing it, I had found my muse for womanhood. I had discovered an energy that would later often come to guide me.

When I encounter a woman who possesses the rare quality of internal radiance, I stop in my tracks. I pause to soak in her wise, soulful essence. In a different way, I sometimes pause to notice those I meet who seem aged beyond their years. Indeed, I have met twenty-somethings who possessed an aged, jaded energy, and I have met souls in their nineties who shine with an energetic, glimmering spirit. These odd and often puzzling differences speak to the concept of *subjective age*, which can be described as the personal experience of feeling old or young, despite chronological age. Research proves that the common aphorism, "You are only as old as you feel," holds truth. An individual's subjective age has been found to have an impact on both physical and psychological well-being. For example, the results of one recent compelling study revealed that individuals' health, behaviors, and longevity are affected by how they perceive their own aging process.[1] Another significant study on subjective age notes that "the age an individual feels is related to changes in characteristic ways of thinking, feeling, and behaving over time."[2] Indeed, the results of these particular studies may be relatively unsurprising (research sometimes only validates that which we instinctively know), for it has been long believed that individuals' attitudes affect the quality and nature of their lives.

This brings us directly back to you, the wonderful woman

reading these pages. What is most important is not your past attitude or behaviors, but how you envision your life from this point forward. Now, this very moment, is your time to refocus and foster an outlook that will serve you to the fullest. It is your attitude that gives you power. For example, older age often gives rises to a list of regrets—of what an individual wishes had been done or not done. Regrets tend to evoke an outlook tinged with thoughts and feelings of blame, guilt, sadness, or anger. The mind's focus turns regretfully to the past and offers no upside, remedy, or learning experience. As a result, these often wholly unproductive thoughts and feelings can unconsciously creep in to create an attitude of hopeless negativity. An individual can subjectively *feel* old and heavy as a result of carrying the burden of inner demons.

The journey ahead will help you find joy and ease through noticing and shifting patterns that do not serve you. Your increased awareness will give you the power of wisdom and choice. If you choose to embrace and nourish an attitude of vibrant positivity, you can create a more joyful life. If you consciously choose to select a subjective age that belies your chronological years, then the years ahead are more likely to be your friend. As always, the choice—the attitude you embrace and enliven—is in your hands. And as it takes no more energy to be positive than negative, you might see the wisdom in embracing the journey into positivity.

The following tips may inspire you to re-evaluate your outlook. They may even inspire you to revamp certain areas of your life. You will notice that some are challenging; trust that your process will lead you to greater self-awareness and positive realizations. Whether the learnings you absorb and the shifts you make are minute or substantial, congratulate yourself for having willingness and courage. You, and only you, can make the greatest difference in your experience of today, your future, and your world. As you begin on this next adventure, give yourself a dose of loving kindness. Remember that you are an amazing, radiant woman. As you acknowledge and let go of what holds you back, your internal light will have the space to shine all the more beautifully and joyfully.

Wisdom Tip 1: Address Any Age-Negative Attitude.

Now is your opportunity to notice if you are being affected or held hostage by an age-negative mindset. Using your journal, write out a list of any age-negative thoughts that come to mind. Setting judgment aside, allow the list to reflect any conscious and unconscious thoughts that begin to arise. For example, your list may include items such as this:

- Younger women are more desirable.
- Younger women are smarter.
- I'm not pretty any longer.
- I can't do what I did in my thirties.
- Older women get fat.
- Women over fifty aren't sexy.
- I don't want to be old.
- I doubt my partner still finds me attractive.
- I am past my prime.
- I can't imagine dating again. What good man would want me at my age?

Once you have completed your list, notice how you feel. Make notes about the feelings and thoughts you've evoked during this exercise. Allow yourself sufficient time and space to appreciate and digest your experience.

Wisdom Tip 2: Create an Age-Positive Attitude.

When you are ready, make a list in your journal that reflects a more age-positive attitude. Although your words may not ring true internally, you may come to adopt a more age-positive attitude in time. Your age-positive list may include thoughts such as these:

- I embrace a joyful, vibrant energy.
- I enjoy each moment of today.
- I enjoy who I am right now.

- I do not wish to be younger than I am today.
- I strive to feel radiant in my body and spirit.
- Chronological age does not define me.
- I am glad to be able to contribute my energy to my community.
- I enjoy giving and sharing with those I love.
- I enjoy my relationship with my partner.
- My retirement allows me to enjoy my days.

Once you have completed your list, notice how you feel. Make notes about the feelings and thoughts you've evoked during this exercise. Allow yourself time and space to appreciate and digest your experience.

Wisdom Tip 3: Craft Your Personal Mantras.

As a result of your age-positive exercise, you may feel more enlivened and aware of your internal gifts and capacities. To encourage a continued, positive mindset, it can be helpful to create a few personal mantras to support your progress.

Mantras are very personal in nature and can be changed as often as you desire. As an example, your first mantra might state: I am a valuable, passionate, resilient woman. Another mantra might note: I love who I am; I am more confident and freer than ever. A third mantra might offer: I am vibrant and beautiful—inside and out.

Whatever your mantras might be, make a few copies to post on your mirror, desk, or refrigerator. Repeat your mantras as proudly and often as possible. The more you repeat your positive mantras, the more positive your outlook will be.

Wisdom Tip 4: Notice the Power of Regret.

This exercise can be a powerful element of your journey. Although positive mantras and age-positive attitudes can be helpful, they don't necessarily eradicate negative thoughts and attitudes that may have formed over time. An individual's regrets often have a silent, negative pull on the psyche, particularly during one's later years. This exercise gives you the opportunity to notice if regrets are negatively affecting your outlook.

Using a fresh page in your journal, allow yourself to write out a list of any regrets you may have. Your list may include items such as the following:

- I regret not going back to school to earn my degree.
- I regret not having children.
- I wish I had never married my husband.
- I wish I had found a life partner.
- I regret not being wilder in my youth.
- I regret having stayed in the same boring job all my life.
- I wish I had done a better job with my children.
- I wish I had mended my relationship with my mother before she died.
- I wish I had been a better daughter.
- I regret not taking advantage of my education to do more with my life.

Whatever your regrets might be, let them surface without judgment. When you have completed your list, make a few notes about whatever thoughts and feelings arise. Make special note of any regrets that can be cured by giving attention to them now or in the future. Mark these regrets with an asterisk.

Now, for a powerful, positive conclusion to this exercise: offset your regrets by noticing whatever gifts appeared as a result of what you didn't do. For example, if you chose one career path over another, notice the gifts that accrued as a result of the path you did choose (e.g., skills accrued, knowledge earned, opportunities embraced, friendships built, financial gain, etc.) Allow yourself time to digest your experience.

Wisdom Tip 5: Write a Disappointment Letter to Yourself.

When you are ready, use your journal to write a compassionate letter of life's disappointments to yourself. This letter can include your list of regrets and whatever other thoughts and feelings arise. The purpose of the letter is to flush out and bring to consciousness any lingering regrets that keep you trapped in blame, sadness, or anger. The following letter offers a brief example:

Dear Wendy,

Regrets! My life is filled with them. I wish I could re-do my life. If I knew back then what I know now, I'd surely have done things differently. I don't even know where to begin.

For starters, I guess I would have stood up for myself more when I was a kid. I wouldn't have let my father push me around. I wouldn't have let myself get bullied at school. I'd have also worked harder in my classes; I didn't take school seriously. I would have taken more risk. I would have tried out for the school plays and the track team. I wouldn't have stayed on the sidelines so much. The list goes on.

I would have done more than dabble in college. I'd have gone on to medical school like I always dreamed. Instead, I got married and lost myself raising my children. I don't regret the kids or the marriage. I regret having lost my own identity.

I regret staying mad at my dad all my life. I was still mad at him when he died. I regret not being with my mom through her cancer. I think I could have done more to let her know she wasn't alone. I regret running from her pain and from my helplessness.

I regret that I'm sixty-five and feel like life has passed me by. I have a good husband, two great kids, and the sweetest grandkids ever. I don't regret them, but I regret that I've

wasted my life. I feel old. I regret not becoming more of who I could have been.
Regretfully,
Wendy

After you have completed your letter, make notes of any thoughts or feelings that arise. Allow yourself time and space to digest this important exercise.

Wisdom Tip 6: Write a Hope-Filled Letter to Yourself.

You now have the opportunity to move away from the regrets that may have held you back in life. Now is the time to be compassionate with yourself. Indeed, the energy spent on regretful thoughts is energy taken away from enjoying the current moment, as well as your future. The purpose of this letter is to channel your energy into a positive, forward-moving realm. Although this positive letter may not ring entirely true at this point, allow yourself to explore your hopes for the future. The following is an example of a hope-filled letter to the self:

Dear Wendy,

The idea of hope makes me smile. I like the idea of thinking about my hopes for the future instead of my regrets. I like the concept of putting my energy into what I can create and change rather than what I've not done.

What do I want for my future? What do I hope to accomplish? I want to volunteer at the hospital. I'd really like to work with cancer patients. I want to read up on cancer—to become more knowledgeable so that I can better help others. I want to take up knitting again. I want to knit scarves and hats for cancer victims.

What else do I hope for? I want to feel better in my body. I want to exercise more. I want to eat better. I want to cook healthy dinners for my husband and me. I want to pull him off the couch and get him to exercise with me. I want to make plans to visit the kids and grandkids at least twice a year.

I am already feeling a little more positive. This feels better than when I was stuck thinking about the past and what I wish I'd done differently. It feels good to turn my energy toward the future. It's uplifting to have a sense of purpose and hope.

Warmly,
Wendy

Wisdom Tip 7: Create a Simple Action Plan.

Armed with the power of your age-positive attitude, personal mantra, and hope-filled ideas, you are ready to move forward. You can now create a simple action plan to help bring your hopes to life.

It is wise to outline small, manageable steps that feel doable. Although it might be tempting to create a plan to fully revamp your life, you will tend to stick with goals that feel easily attainable. In addition, you will be more likely to continue on your path when you can see steady results.

As the goal of this exercise is to give yourself the gift of positive reinforcement, keep your action plan simple, focused, and specific. For example, Wendy's action plan might read:

- Start walking for twenty minutes a day, three times per week. Begin this weekend.
- Research, before the weekend, the starting date of the next free community center class on eating and cooking healthfully. Enroll in the next class that is available.
- Find my box of knitting supplies in the attic. Knit a fun scarf within thirty days.
- Research online courses in cancer education; enroll in a course within forty-five days.
- Research volunteer opportunities at the hospital. Take the necessary steps to apply within ninety days.

As you move forward with a positive, can-do attitude, your life will begin to take on a different flavor. You will, in fact, slowly but surely begin to radiate a different energy. As you cast aside self-ageism, you will shift your internal world. In this way, you will begin to alter the hold of ageism in the greater world. You may not notice yourself changing; the shifts may be quite imperceptible to you at first. Trust, however, that you will become more of who you want to be with every step you take forward in the name of your own joy-filled womanhood.

And I thank you, from the very bottom of my heart, for having the desire and courage to fan your inner light. Thank you for wanting to shine with powerful, ageless beauty—to radiate as you are truly meant to do.

CHAPTER 2

Loving Your Maturing Self from the Inside Out

*L*et me introduce you to a client I'll call "A Woman over a Certain Age." As she sat in my office, her words of dismay and irritation filled the room. She noted with disgust, "I can't *stand* my body. I absolutely *hate* the way I look. Worse yet, I think I am starting not to like myself. It's awful. I don't know where to start because it feels like *everything* is going downhill. I don't fit into clothes like I did even ten years ago. I don't expect to look like I'm twenty, but do I have to look like *this?* My skin has age spots and wrinkles. The lines around my eyes make me look 100 years old.

"My hair is thinning—even my eyebrows are fading away! Believe it or not, I have to see my hairstylist almost twice a month just to cover my grays! It's ridiculous. The upkeep, the sheer maintenance to look half-decent, is so time consuming and expensive.

No matter what I do, Botox or whatever, I *feel* old. No skin cream or facial is going to do the trick. I'm way past that. And, I swear, from the loose, creepy skin on my arms to spider veins on my legs, I'm embarrassed to put on anything but shapeless pants and long-sleeved shirts. Forget wearing clothes that fit closely, because the extra rolls around my waistline ooze over no matter how much I exercise. It's just not fair. I eat right, exercise, and still have a spare tire? *Really?*

"Oh, and don't get me going on my boobs. Saggy doesn't even begin to describe my once-perky breasts—seriously, I had awesome boobs twenty or thirty years ago. Until they find a treatment that can tighten and lift my eyes, jowls, breasts, belly, and thighs, I might as well wear a paper bag over my entire body."

I listened quietly, and I understood her dismay. This woman is not alone in her frustration. Most women—if not *every* woman—might be able to empathize with her irritation and her pain.

Let's move forward with a little experiment. Pause for a moment to take a look in the mirror. Whether you find yourself peering at your reflection in your bathroom, bedroom, office, or store dressing room, do you *like* the woman you see? Now pause to notice if you *love* the woman who looks back at you. As you look into a mirror, notice if your mind takes you straight into a critical evaluation of those gray hairs, wrinkles, stretch marks, looser skin, and age spots. Notice if you orient your eyes toward the physical, age-related aspects of the woman you are. Perhaps you find yourself staring at your naked form, fuming at the toll of gravity and time. Yet if you happen to focus on the warm light in your eyes, the loving glow of your smile, or the empowered lift within your heart space, you are connecting with other aspects of the woman before you. This eternally ageless woman—this gorgeous inner being—is always waiting for you. Sometimes, however, she is hidden behind layers of ageism, fears, and wounds. If you're game, let's bring this woman out for some rejuvenation and play.

Now, stay in front of that mirror and give that gorgeous woman in front of you a kiss. Plant a big lipstick (or no lipstick) kiss on that mirror. Remember this moment, for it is evidence of love and play. That kiss, and the thousands to come, are important to that precious woman in the mirror. She deserves each and every heart-felt kiss that comes her way.

Now, take a step back and look at the woman in front of you once again. She is a true work of art, isn't she? If you're in the mood (or not yet in the mood), perhaps dance and twirl like a little girl. Smile. Giggle. Sing if you like. Immerse yourself in the moment, letting go of your busy mind. Give yourself a warm hug. Now look in the mirror again. Notice how you feel and how you look. If you let your inner child come out to play, you might notice a sweet radiance and a sense of childlike delight. You might notice that you feel lighter and freer. This is your eternal radiance in action. From this little experiment, you now might know that you can capture that lovely, pure energy any time of the day or night. We might not be able to prevent the body from aging, but the mind and spirit—your true, inner self—can be ageless.

You might find yourself saying dryly, "Thanks for the cute experiment, but it's not very helpful on a day-to-day level."

I would smile, give you a hug, and say, "Oh, I understand. Yet have a little faith. Positive actions breed positive thoughts, and positive thoughts breed positive actions. If you laugh in the face of ageism, you might just find your wise and playful inner child staring back at you."

Although the above experiment was small and simple, it might have given you an idea of the power of your own attitude. If you focus on wrinkles and the other age-related barnacles that life brings, then that's what you'll see. If you focus on your vibrant being as a whole—the brilliant essence of all that you are and all that you've embraced in life—then luminosity is what you'll see.

If you are willing, my friend, this chapter will help you make this idea come to life. You'll find tips and tools to bring this concept into action in your daily life. As you move forward, you'll begin to breathe greater life into your precious and powerful eternal radiance.

A Mental and Emotional Facelift

Indeed, there may be times that you don't readily recognize yourself as the woman you see in a photograph or mirror. I've sometimes caught a glimpse of myself in a photo and said, "That doesn't look like me!" This makes perfect sense, for we often hold mental images of ourselves as we were in our earlier years. The brain, it seems, sometimes gets stuck in a time-warp that makes a current image seem incongruent with certain visions held in one's memory. The contrast and juxtaposition of these images is normal, yet we tend to judge one image as being better or worse than the other. It's important to remember that all of the images are wonderful; it's the critical mind that gets us into trouble by saying, "Oh, you *used* to be so pretty! You don't look like that any longer! Now you look old, worn, and saggy." Your critical voice might continue endlessly on, telling you that you are fat, wrinkly, gray, or other negative words that come to mind. The mind likes to busy itself with often harsh, unkind labels and comparisons.

Of course, we can't deny the aging process; in fact, there's no upside to avoiding the obvious truth of life's wear and tear on the body. We can, however, learn to use the mind rather than letting the mind use (and often torture) the self. Although the mind can get busy and even quite mean at any stage in life, it can become especially critical and judgmental as we age.

Given our youth-oriented culture, it can be especially difficult to escape the collective mantra that often says, "Being young (or looking young) is everything. Youth is beautiful. Run from old age. Run as fast as you can from those depressing, worthless, ugly years." In fact, your work in chapter 1 may have helped you notice and reframe your own age-negative thoughts and attitudes. You may even hear a fresh new voice saying, "I am stronger and tougher now than ever. I find myself—and my life—more beautiful every day. I've been working a lifetime to get to this place of loving who I am." You, indeed, may have noticed that your mind is a very powerful thing. As you move forward, you will continue to build on the awareness you've been generating.

To foster your age-positive energy and wisdom, let's get a bit negative in a purposeful, honest way. In truth, it's important to look at the downside of aging. It's vital that we honestly explore the feelings of denial, anger, fear, anxiety, embarrassment, depression, sadness, and hopelessness that sometimes creep in as we are faced with aging issues. These uncomfortable feelings (and so many more) can take over if we are blind to their pull and power. Yet if we face such issues with wise awareness, we can come to make friends with these forces. Indeed, inside each one of these feelings lies a message that will help you embrace your aging process with joy and power.

Remember this truth: That which you learn to acknowledge, honor, and *release when necessary* loses its power to control you. That which you come to accept and embrace becomes a powerful source of support for you.

Wisdom Tip 8: Ponder the Disadvantages of Aging.

Purposefully focus on the downside of aging. When you are ready, close your eyes to allow yourself to imagine and experience the feelings that arise when you think of the negative elements of aging. Give attention to any feelings that surface. Notice, too, if any thoughts come to you. When you are ready, open your eyes.

With an open, nonjudgmental attitude, make a list of the feelings that arose. Also make notes regarding any thoughts that came to you. Notice, however, that this particular journey is oriented more to the exploration of your feelings rather than your thoughts. Close your eyes for a moment and then return your focus to your list of feelings. Notice how this review of your list makes you feel. Do you feel lighter, heavier, sad, happy, anxious, irritated, angry, or some other feeling? Make simple notes about whatever you observe.

As you scan your list of thoughts, pause to consider this: Do you want to accept the thoughts you listed as being factual? Is it necessary or valuable for you to accept these particular "downsides"? Allow yourself to consider these questions; make any notes that feel important to you.

Wisdom Tip 9: Focus on "Charged" Feelings.

Without judgment, take another look at your list of feelings. Using a scale of 0–10 (with "0" being the lowest impact and "10" being the highest), rate the power that each feeling has over you. For example, if two of the feelings you noted were "sad" and "terrified," you might place a "5" next to "sad" and a "9" next to "terrified." Such self-ratings would indicate that you feel moderately sad and extremely terrified about aging.

Allow yourself to notice without judgment which items are more emotionally and mentally charged for you (the higher the number, the greater the charge). Honor these feelings; they are yours to notice and feel. Make notes as you desire.

Wisdom Tip 10: Describe Your Feelings.

On a fresh page, write out each feeling word you listed. Leave several free lines after each word. Then write a sentence that describes what that feeling means to you. There is no "right" or "wrong" way to do this exercise; just follow your natural intuition. For example, if the word "fearful" is on your list, you might note, "I feel fearful that I will be a burden to my family if serious health issues arise." As another example, if "excited" appears on your list, you might write, "I feel tremendously excited to explore new aspects of my life after retirement." Feel free to write more than one descriptive sentence for each feeling. Make any notes that feel appropriate to you.

Wisdom Tip 11: Allow Time for a Feeling-Oriented Reflection.

Pause to reflect on both the feelings and thoughts that arose during this important exercise; make notes about your process. You have now explored the realm where the mind and body connect—the world of your feelings.

I applaud you for having the courage to face your aging-related feelings openly and honestly. This isn't necessarily comfortable or easy work. In fact, it can be downright tough. It's important to foster faith in your inner power. Remember, the more you face the negative pull of your fears and worries, the more you will be freed from their toxic energy.

As you continue to work toward building an age-positive attitude, notice that your age-negative patterns can be utilized to further your progress. Although this concept might seem unfamiliar, remember that there is often a hidden upside to even the most negative-appearing force. When we take the time to slow down, to really dissect our presuppositions, attitudes, and feelings, we can discover the kernels of wise, truthful energy that usually wait below the surface. Our very fears and worries often hold the most vital keys to our freedom. In fact, once we take a look at our fears and harness them to take action, there is often a reduction in feelings such as anxiety, depression, and hopelessness. Trust that every step you take—the little ones and the big ones—will work in concert to create positive energy in your life.

Wisdom Tip 12: Create Positive Energy.

Return to your previous exercise for just a moment, pausing at *Wisdom Tip 10*. Notice each descriptive sentence that you wrote. Now write out a proactive goal, positive message, or growth opportunity that could result from the original descriptive sentence. Let each new sentence reflect a positive, can-do attitude. Although the shifts may seem minor to you, simply focus on the positive energy and the upside potential.

Using the example above, "I feel fearful that I will be a burden to my family if serious health issues arise," a proactive goal might note, "I will take my physician's advice to eat a heart-healthy diet. I will do the necessary grocery shopping and meal planning this weekend." A second proactive goal might note, "I will investigate long-term care insurance. I will apply for an affordable policy within two weeks."

Follow this process for every descriptive sentence you wrote in the above exercise.

Wisdom Tip 13: Notice How Positive Messages Make You Feel.

As you review your positive statements, notice how each sentence makes you feel. Again, even if the shift or goal seems minor, allow yourself to notice any fresh, positive feelings that arise. Write out a list of your positive feelings, even if they seem relatively faint. For example, you might feel slightly hopeful or mildly refreshed. You also might feel invigorated, powerful, or tremendously energized. If negative energy wants to creep in, gently acknowledge it before returning your focus to your positive feelings.

Wisdom Tip 14: Nurture Your Positive Feelings.

Feed your positive feelings by paying attention to them. We often pay far too much attention to our negative feelings and far too little attention to the positive feelings that want to peek through like sunshine through heavy clouds. Write out each positive feeling and a related can-do message on a sticky note.

For example, you might write, "Hopeful! I feel hopeful about my health when I know I am eating right!" Another note might state, "Energized! Positive, goal-oriented actions keep me feeling vibrant, energized, and excited about life!"

Place your positive messages where you will see them often; these positive messages will feed your mind and spirit.

Attitude Is (Nearly) Everything

It's likely very clear to you by now that much of this journey into aging with power and grace focuses on the theme of one's personal attitude toward life. This concept is so important to embrace and emphasize throughout your life (and thus, throughout the pages of this book), for your attitude is where you hold your greatest power in life. Sadly, I have seen far too many souls turn dark and withered as a result of life-long negative thought patterns and behaviors. It is not a person's level of physical attractiveness, wealth, or external power that ultimately matters; it is attitude that makes every difference in long run.

When I think of the incredible power that attitude has in determining certain outcomes in life, a certain wild-eyed sixty-four-year-old woman comes to mind. This energetic client, Anna, typically saunters into my office with muddy hiking boots and an untucked flannel shirt. Grayhaired and of round, stocky build, this lovely woman might be a farmer, a skier, a mountain climber, or a baker. In fact, she is all of those things and more. In her not-too-distant past, she was also an IT executive in a fast-paced major city. Yet all of these descriptions can't begin to define Anna. Indeed, what you notice most about Anna is her adventurous, almost childlike, way of being. To be in proximity to Anna is to feel a maelstrom of fire, whimsy, intelligence, and curiosity. Anna truly has a most powerful and joyful way of embracing life.

Following a quick divorce from her philandering first husband, Anna ignored her pain and turned her significant energy into her career. Her career became her greatest passion, and she immersed herself in the business world for over three solid decades. Anna also took to traveling around the globe when the opportunity arose; her whirlwind journeys gave her life greater depth and adventure.

When retirement came, Anna was not ready to slow down. With new and old hobbies vying for attention, Anna found herself busier than ever. She then suddenly found herself contemplating remarriage. A skiing accident temporarily sidelined Anna, but it also brought romance into her life. At age sixty-eight, Anna found herself knee-deep in an implausible relationship with Ted, a farmer she met during a physical therapy appointment. She found him charming and delightful until the good-hearted man began to move emotionally closer to her. Anna found herself confused and she began to withdraw. She fled to a mountain nearly halfway around the world, but she found no real respite or solutions in her retreat. With no career to distract her, Anna found herself face-to-face with all of Anna—her unresolved history, her triumphs, and her lows.

In our first appointments together, Anna slowly offered intimate segments of her tale. Despite her effervescent exterior, the realm of emotions was not Anna's forte. It was the combination of Anna's words, eyes, gestures, and tone of voice that revealed her inner world. Anna laughed as she pulled at a frayed edge of her shirt and said, "This thing is as old as the hills—as old and worn as me!"

When I smiled and asked how she was faring, her energy faded as she noted, "Ted wants to get married. I'm too old for that. I've been there, over forty years ago, I can't do that again. Mixing finances and households at this late age? Better to stay safe and single! Who needs the pain?"

Anna paused, and a childish light came into her eyes. With renewed enthusiasm she uttered, "I have to say, though, that I love his charm and his playfulness. I love his honesty. He's a widower—married for nearly forty years. Seriously, it's the whole white-picket-fence-front-porch-swing-tomato-garden-cows-and-chickens-in-the-yard thing. I know he's a good bet. He's a good man. And I can see myself with him until . . ." Anna paused again as a flash of pain darkened her eyes and she tapped her foot. "This is what I need help on. I've told you that my first husband was a real jerk. He cheated on me. He abandoned me. He wasn't a great choice. I ran, but I didn't forget."

Anna sighed, and her eyes softened as she said, "If I could somehow let that hurt go and move forward, I think I'd be a great sixty-eight-year-old wife. There's a lot of life left in this old girl. I don't feel like I'm sixty-eight inside. Part of me thinks that it would be great to share my life with Ted. He loves me—flabby jowls, drooping boobs, elephant skin, and all. He likes the kid in me, and I like the kid in him."

Her eyes clouded over. "But what if I'm too old for this? What if he decides I'm too lumpy or wrinkly? What if I get ill—cancer or something—and he bolts on me?" Anna shook her head and half-smiled. Her eyes lit up again and she chuckled. "This is hard for me to say, but I really love him. He's a good man. When I'm with him, I feel like I'm a kid again—no matter what my body says. We're like two nine-year-old kids together, just playing and exploring. I know we're a good fit—Ted and me. I think that maybe I just need help getting out of my own way."

Indeed, Anna's inner child, ever hopeful and filled with enthusiasm, was a bit at war with the closed-off, jaded side of her being. The outcome was within Anna's own control. Filled with oodles of intelligence, energy, and power, Anna could do as she pleased.

Aspects of Anna's story may resonate with you on several levels. You might be reminded of unresolved psychological wounds that hold you back. You might find yourself thinking that you feel older (or younger) than your physical age. Anna's situation reminds us that it is often psychological factors—both mental and emotional—that affect us far more deeply than chronological age. Indeed, in the course of Anna's appointments, there were times that I surely saw her ten-year-old self come to life. Then other times, particularly when she struggled with the hurt of betrayal and abandonment, a very old, embittered energy took hold. Anna courageously wrestled to bring her ageless, powerful wisdom into communion with her willing, childlike enthusiasm.

Anna looked inside herself to determine what she wanted in her future. She worked to dismantle the fears that impeded her forward movement. Anna found that most of her fears were imaginary and that many were unconscious blockages against intimacy. The fears that were substantive were few. Anna accessed her inner courage and began to make shifts necessary to create the life she wanted. She continued her self-work through journaling and psychotherapy sessions as needed. As well, the pragmatic issues that needed attention were outlined, plans were made, and specific goals were set. Each item was addressed with wise planning and careful attention. Although the process was not simple or quick, Anna moved forward step-by-step. Her journey was not a singular event; *it was a process* of millions of miniscule events, years of curious searching, and a lifetime of secret yearning.

Throughout the journey, Anna's caution and willing energy were met by Ted's genuine, patient support. In the end, wild-eyed Anna chose to undertake an adventure into love. She chose to shift away from hurt and fear and into a space of new possibilities. Indeed, I had the delightful opportunity to see the radiant pair together. I can tell you that one young-at-heart sixty-eight-year-old and one spry seventy-year-old made for a most wonderful, spirited couple. Had Anna chosen to let negative fears run her life (fear of hurt, fear of aging, and fear of what the future might hold), her world would surely be different.

Perhaps there are areas in your own life that are held back by similar fears. You may be in a place where you feel interested in change. You might be ready to explore the idea of shaking off those constraints—those doubts and fears—and moving forward into a new way of thinking and a new way of being. You can create whatever change you desire. It's so simple, and yet extraordinarily tough, to manifest change. You might want to place a copy of this next Wisdom Tip in your back pocket, on your wall, or at your desk—for it is basic, powerful, and true.

Wisdom Tip 15: Generate Empowered Change.

Change is easy, and change is tough. Change happens whether you want it or not. That being said, it makes sense to step up and be the director of your own life whenever possible. Change is easier to understand, accept, and control when you face it with power, wisdom, and grace. As you practice the following nine basic "Steps for Empowered Change," you'll meet life's many challenges and changes with greater ease.

Nine Steps for Empowered Change

1. Engage in the necessary inner exploration to become aware of what you truly want in life. Use whatever methods help you broaden your horizons—journaling, sharing with others, or researching opportunities.
2. Foster a forward-thinking, growth-oriented mindset. If you find yourself getting stuck in the past, strive to shift toward what the future holds for you.
3. Investigate what is holding you back. Journal and reflect to understand your specific fears or limiting life circumstances.
4. Seek outside support whenever needed. Whether you consult a friend, business professional, or psychotherapist, there is great strength and wisdom in obtaining support when needed.
5. Access the courage to make shifts by continually acknowledging that you have the bravery and power to create positive change in your life.
6. Create simple, specific goals to help you move forward with purpose and clarity. Main goals can seem more doable when supported by achievable microgoals.
7. Utilize your amazing energy to follow through. The energy you previously invested in other areas (doing for others, focusing on the past, etc.) is now readily available and can be channeled to create positive change.
8. Call upon your patience as you progress. Be kind to yourself, for change doesn't manifest overnight.
9. Congratulate yourself for every micro-step forward. Remember that your journey is a process, not a singular event.

The above concept—this nine-step schema for empowered change—is so important that you may notice it woven into various elements of the journey ahead. In true pyramid fashion, key concepts will help you build a strong foundation that will support future work. The concepts you embrace will become so familiar that you will find yourself naturally viewing your life (and any changes you desire to make) with a more positive, empowered mindset.

The Power of Self-Esteem

There is no magic pill or singular trick for creating a positive mindset, but a mixture of willingness and strong self-esteem is a powerful potion. To more fully appreciate the importance of self-esteem, it's important to understand the nature of self-esteem. As many people use the terms "self-esteem" and "self-confidence" interchangeably, it's important to first address the differences between the two terms.

Self-confidence tends to arise from feeling competent in a certain arena or as a result of having a particular attribute. Self-confidence is often based on more superficial characteristics or qualities; if the sources of self-confidence are decreased or absent, a drop in self-confidence will result. By its very nature, self-confidence tends to fluctuate based upon a variety of factors, including external events, abilities, and perceptions. Common sources of self-confidence include physical appearance, employment, material acquisitions, and achievements.

The following examples offer insight into the wide-ranging, sometimes transitory nature of self-confidence. A person who is focused on physical appearance may derive a sense of self-confidence from the image in the mirror. One's profession may also be a source of self-confidence. An individual's hobbies, such as sports, cooking, and creative arts, may be sources of self-confidence. A student may feel self-confident in respect to certain school subjects or extracurricular achievements. A materialistic person may feel self-confident when wearing the latest clothes, driving an expensive "look at what I drive" car, or owning the priciest gadgets. Interestingly, a person whose self-confidence arises purely from external factors may appear to be highly self-confident, yet they may be severely lacking in self-esteem. As well, although self-confidence may contribute to self-esteem, one's sense of self-esteem is far more widereaching.

When it comes to self-esteem, an individual's overall sense of self-worth is the focus. In essence, a person's level of self-esteem tends to reflect the individual's core, overarching sense of personal value. Self-esteem generally stems from two arenas: an individual's sense of self-worth, coupled with the individual's perception of being valued by others. Given that an individual's personal perceptions give rise to the sense of self-esteem, the concept of self-esteem is clearly subjective in nature; a person's sense of self-esteem does not necessarily reflect an objective evaluation of the individual or the manner in which others see or value the individual. Although the self-esteem aspect of an individual's personality is generally enduring, it may shift over time depending upon significant life events and circumstances. For example, an individual who grew up in an unloving, critical home environment may have very low self-esteem. Yet with concerted self-work, that individual may come to develop and nurture a deep sense of self-respect and self-worth.

Self-esteem is built—and is truly earned—as a result of self-work. As a wonderful friend noted, "Self-esteem is a muscle we build—just as we build resilience in life. Like abdominal muscles, self-esteem is the core of our emotional posture. We sometimes take it for granted (just like our body's core muscles) until we end up suffering from not working to keep it strong." Whereas physical muscles are built by physical activity, the muscle of self-esteem is built by actively living your life in accord with your personal standards. *Self-esteem can be fostered and strengthened by consistently holding yourself to the ideals that support you in being the best version of yourself.* Through this lens, self-esteem can be seen as a quality that is accessible to every person who desires to nurture and strengthen this vital, powerful force.

Individuals with a strong sense of self-esteem tend to genuinely like and appreciate themselves. Although those with a strong sense of self-esteem may have occasional, natural periods of self-doubt, their sense of self-worth does not tend to depend on external circumstances, material possessions, and approval from others. Those with lower self-esteem may tend to question their personal value; they may feel unworthy, unlovable, or somehow defective. They secretly (or not-so-secretly) dislike who they are. Poor self-esteem tends to manifest in many areas of life. Those with lower self-esteem also tend to struggle with self-respect and may exhibit less respect for others. Of course, lower levels of self-esteem may also give rise to people-pleasing tendencies, self-deprecating attitudes, and a wide variety of other unhealthy behaviors. When low self-esteem is at work, an individual may increasingly feel unworthy, stuck, and hopeless. Yet when an individual begins to work on self-esteem issues, positive and long-lasting changes can result.

As you may now realize, your sense of self-esteem is an incredibly significant force in your life. Self-esteem has been found to affect many important areas of life, including success in social relationships, mental health, physical health, work, and education.[1] This is not surprising, for your sense of self-esteem is foundational. Self-esteem impacts your daily life because it reflects (consciously and unconsciously) how you feel and think about yourself, as well as how you believe others perceive and value you. All of your self-perceptions—both the positive and the negative—work together to form your sense of self-esteem. When you consider self-esteem from this vantage point, its power to impact your life is astounding.

It is a blessing that strong self-esteem can be cultivated and fostered throughout life. There is great power to be had in knowing that you have the power to increase your level of self-esteem. The process of self-esteem building is a journey that requires your wise participation. Your self-esteem will slowly grow as you become more aware of and attuned to your needs, your desires, and your values. Your self-esteem will flourish steadily when you consciously strive to live as your best self, turning natural stumbles into learning opportunities. By knowing and standing in your truth—by honoring yourself, your moral code, and all that is important to you—your self-esteem will become ever more powerful. *Your self-esteem will expand and shine as you practice being your own best self.*

If you have excellent self-esteem, you're blessed to have nurtured (and earned) this vital quality. If not, do not worry; self-esteem can be built. Whether your level of self-esteem is extremely low or in a more moderate range, you truly can increase your sense of self-worth. The overarching self-esteem goal for every one of us might be this:

I will build a strong sense of self-esteem that allows me to move through life with a deep inner sense of self-worth and self-respect. I will honor the truth that self-esteem does not stem from or rely upon physicality, external qualities, material possessions, or other transitory elements. I will be patient with myself as I learn how to cultivate true self-esteem. I will learn to know my truth and stand in my truth. Regardless of the opinions of others, I will stand up for and honor the woman I am. I will be flexible enough to bend and learn, yet I will not yield at the expense of my values and self-respect. I will learn from my stumbles as I strive to be my best self. I will love, respect, and value others . . . as I love, respect, and value myself.

If you think you are past your prime and that your self-esteem has nowhere to go but down, take heart. Research indicates that self-esteem actually *peaks* at age sixty. After age sixty, self-esteem then remains at a constant level until age seventy, and then declines only slightly through age ninety.[1] It is absolutely thrilling to offer you the above research findings, for these statistics offer a lovely reminder that mature age surely has its benefits.

Indeed, there is great comfort to be had in knowing that the earlier decades of life, often spent creating a sense of identity and struggling through one maturation crisis after another, are behind us. And for those who are blooming a little bit later in life, it's reassuring to know that there's plenty of time remaining to build a strong sense of self-esteem. So no matter your age, I say, "You go, girl. Forget about your chronological age. There's no better time than now to create the woman—and the life—of your dreams."

Let me introduce you to Bess, a diffident woman in her sixties. Preferring to dress in tidy, shapeless clothing that hung in folds over her small frame, Bess seemed to seek invisibility. In fact, Bess once noted, "I've always liked staying in the background. I've been the mousey, quiet one my entire life. But since my husband died, I realized that I can either wither away into nothingness or make a fresh start. As hard as it is for me to get out of my shell, I want to build some confidence. I want to know who I am. I was a kindergarten teacher years ago, but I've not done much with my life other than that. I'm not really good at anything besides being a housewife. I wasn't able to have children, so my husband was everything to me. The value of my life was in being a good wife and caretaker.

"When my husband died—cancer took him after a long battle—my life became empty and unimportant. My sister is worried about me; she thinks I am stuck in grief and not moving forward after my husband's death. She says I'm getting depressed and is insistent that I get some support. So, here I am. I figure I'll give this 'moving forward' thing a try."

It took Bess a great deal of courage to reach out for support, to move out of the comfort zone of the world she had known for over forty years. Yet, slowly and surely, Bess moved through her significant fears to discover what a new future might hold for her. Among other issues, Bess discovered that she suffered from low self-esteem. For an incredibly long time, Bess's sole identity was that of a wife and caregiver. When those roles disappeared, Bess's sense of self nearly disappeared along with them. So the work began to discover a new Bess (or perhaps a hidden Bess) who had desires, needs, strengths, and values that were waiting to be explored and grown.

Although Bess had "no idea" who she was, it became clear after several sessions that Bess had quite a lot to offer herself and the world. As we delved into her history, I found that there was much more to timid Bess than met the eye. Bess, as it turned out, was an extremely skilled seamstress and quilter. She was also a fabulous baker with a special knack for creating breads and hearty muffins. Bess's cooking talents also shone in the realm of creating home-made jellies and honeys.

I said to Bess in the midst of one session, "You're quite a remarkable woman, aren't you?"

"Oh, no," she responded with genuine humility. "It's all really nothing. My husband got such joy out of providing for me that he didn't want me to work, so I just had time on my hands. I put my time to use, that's all."

Although Bess was confident in her abilities—she knew she was highly capable at sewing, cooking, baking, cleaning, and even attending to the basic mechanics of running a household—she did not realize that she was valuable beyond the skillset she had brought to her husband and home life. Indeed, much to her sur-prise, Bess eventually came to find that some of the skills she had honed during her years as a wife and homemaker were quite valu-able in the outside world.

With much courage and effort, Bess began to explore herself on many levels. She became more attuned to her skills and capa-bilities. She also began to appreciate the tasks within her skillset that gave her joy and those that were more lackluster. Bess dipped her toes in the business world. Bess enrolled in several market-ing and business courses at the local junior college. Despite her fears of "being too old," she passed her classes with ease. This step, and every other step forward she took, increased her self-esteem. Now armed with confidence in her new knowledge and the power of a bit more self-esteem, Bess turned her attention to what she came to honor as an exceptionally strong creative ability. With an abundance of time before her, Bess could spend her time however she liked.

Ultimately, Bess decided to put her efforts into the arenas that gave her the most joy—quilting and making honey. Initially with her sister at her side for moral support, Bess made inquiries, discovering that a few local stores were delighted to carry her home-made honey. She also found that several gift stores in the county were thrilled to offer her exquisite quilts for sale. Several months later, Bess was asked to teach quilting classes. Step by step and day by day, Bess began to explore a bigger world. In this process of working through what frightened her, Bess became stronger. By tuning in to her desires—to what gave her joy—Bess came to know what she wanted out of life. As a result of taking action to create what she wanted (by moving forward with focus and intention), Bess came to feel her power. Over time, Bess—an increasingly not-so-timid Bess—came to see and appreciate more of who she was.

Within two years of her husband's passing, Bess found herself busier and with a stronger sense of self than ever. As the "new" Bess said with a thoughtful smile, "I loved my husband so much that I honestly can't say that I am happier now. I miss him every day. But I can say that I feel better about myself—about who I am as a whole person. I feel much stronger and aware of my capacities. Although I was happy in the shelter of my marriage, my growth as a woman was stunted in many ways—stunted because of the closed nature of my life. Now my happiness is built on many things, like new connections, a stronger sense of myself, and an odd feeling that my life is just beginning in many ways. For a sixty-seven-year-old, it seems a strange thing to say."

I had to smile. For a once-sheltered sixty-seven-year-old woman, it seemed like a most tremendous thing to say. Bess's delightful trajectory was not a result of fate or serendipity. Bess could have remained mired in grief and loss. Instead, she *chose* to heed her sister's wise urgings. She *chose* to seek support to move forward so she could create a life that was fulfilling and positive. Bess *chose* to summon her courageous spirit to adapt to the changes and foster the possibilities that life brought her way.

Bess didn't let age get in her way; instead, she utilized the skills she had accrued throughout her life to build a new, strong sense of self and a fresh, lovely life that gave her a different kind of joy.

Normalizing and Addressing Key Mental Health Concerns: Emotions, Depression, Anxiety, and More

It's vitally important to be honest about mental health issues such as depression, anxiety, and chronic stress. I cringe at our culture's tendency to minimize, marginalize, or even hide mental health concerns. This flabbergasts me, for mental health issues are a part of life. Just like childhood tantrums, adolescent acne, broken bones, and cancer, psychological difficulties are a normal (if unwanted) part of humanity. So why pretend they don't exist? Why cover up our hurts with too many anti-depressants, anti-anxiety pills, and tranquilizing substances? Of course, medications are absolutely essential for millions of individuals—and they are a key component of psychological treatment for many—yet it is of concern that psychotherapy is often ignored or devalued as a necessary component in the treatment process. And in the cases of necessary psychopharmacological treatment, why is there an onus on the use of necessary medications? Wouldn't it make sense to honor the need for an anti-anxiety medication just as we honor the need for blood pressure medication?

Clearly, it's time that we normalize mental health issues. It's well past time to advocate for and welcome psychotherapy as a necessary component in the treatment of anxiety, depression, stress, trauma, and the other mental health issues that leave many suffering in embarrassed silence. And it's certainly time to understand psychopharmacology better and to encourage wise usage of medication to allow for greater natural joy in life. You can be a part of positive change by taking your mental health concerns seriously, by advocating for proper care, and by standing up for what you need. There is no need to suffer in silence or to be embarrassed if you're depressed, anxious, stressed, or fearful—you *deserve* to be supported if you are hurting inside.

Although mental health issues in the later decades of life often share similar threads with other life stages, the more mature life phases do have their own unique challenges. An individual's later years can involve a great many changes that often include children leaving home, change in marital status, death of a spouse, retirement, altered social relationships, and the decline and loss of parents. Many individuals are also impacted by shifts in finances, general health concerns, and a slow change in physical abilities. These significant changes often take a cumulative, heavy toll on the psyche.

Given our culture's "just get through it" mentality, many women are simply unaware that these myriad changes can have long-term psychological effects. The changes that life brings are often gradual in nature; they creep in over time, often in imperceptible ways. With busy lives filled with to-do lists that are often focused on making ends meet or caring for others, the challenges of life are often readily addressed, yet the toll on the psyche is often dismissed, marginalized, or altogether ignored. As a result, it is not surprising that many women "suddenly" notice that they feel depressed or chronically stressed. It's no wonder that so many women "wake up one day" feeling anxious and in need of "something" to help them feel rejuvenated or make life easier to bear.

Your emotions have a message. Your feelings—all of them—matter. Although I often emphasize the importance of maintaining and fanning one's deep, inner sense of joy throughout life and the challenges it brings, it is also important to notice and honor other emotions as they arise. It's not normal (or even possible) for any person to be 100 percent "happy" all the time. Strangely, our culture often gives the message that we "should" *always* be happy and that something is wrong if we are not. This is a ridiculous idea. Human beings have a wide range of feelings at their disposal; all of them are important, not just one or two of them. So whether you notice that you are feeling angry, sad, fearful, disgusted, or joyful, allow yourself to appreciate the emotion and the underlying message. If you strive to ignore or push away your uncomfortable emotions, they will only hide and percolate.

If you find yourself getting chronically "stuck" in a certain emotion such as anger or sadness, it's important to notice if certain emotions are controlling you. You'll observe that you feel more powerful when you pause to notice your emotions and then make the choice to use your emotional energy wisely.

Wisdom Tip 16: Take Compassionate Control of Your Emotional Energy.

The following "Steps for Emotional Empowerment" may be helpful in allowing you to notice, regulate, and beneficially utilize your emotions—particularly those that tend to "get a hold on you." By making friends with your emotions, you'll feel more in touch and empowered. Although the steps below are directed at noticing one emotion at a time, it's important to note that more than one emotion may surface at once. When you are working with more than one emotion, slow down to allow yourself to thoroughly process each emotion.

Steps for Emotional Empowerment

1. Pause to notice when you get "hit" by a strong or hurtful emotion. Breathe slowly.
2. Notice the sensations in your body (short breaths, racing heart, flushed face).
3. Identify and name the emotion (sadness, anger, fear, etc.). Breathe slowly.
4. Notice the sensations and emotion in your body once again; allow yourself to feel the emotion, then allow it to *move*.
5. Express to yourself (or others as appropriate) how you feel by saying, "I feel angry," "I feel scared," "I feel hurt," "I feel criticized," "I feel worried," "I feel sad," etc.

6. Engage in a gentle activity, such as walking, stretching, or yoga. Breathe.
7. Notice how you feel (tired, weary, spent, energized, etc.) and attend to yourself with a supportive, self-soothing behavior (meditating, taking a shower, drinking tea, etc.).
8. Journal about your feelings without any judgment. Allow yourself to express and "vent" your emotions freely and without concern for grammar or form.

As you get to know your emotions better and become more accustomed to all of the feelings that are a natural part of your humanity, you will feel more at ease with yourself. By not judging any emotion as "bad" or "good," you will come to find that every emotion has a message that wants to be heard and valued. For example, if you feel sad and have the urge to cry, remember that your tears have a message, be it pain, disappointment, or sorrow. Your tears are allowing you to feel, express, and cleanse your inner hurt. As another example, if you are angry as a result of feeling disrespected by a loved one, your anger has a purpose. Your anger wants to be noticed and honored. Your anger may carry a message that asks you to clearly state your feelings and take action to set clear, respectful boundaries.

When your emotions are felt rather than repressed or devalued, you will be more in touch with your inner power. In time, you will not fear being ruled or overtaken by any particular emotion. You will feel empowered by knowing that you are in charge of your emotional responses. Whether you are feeling angry, irritated, or anxious, you will find that you need not let your emotional responses take charge of you.

The Cloud of Depression

Although attitude isn't everything when it comes to depression, research shows that your outlook on the aging process may impact your risk for major depression. Once again utilizing the concept of subjective age (i.e., how individuals experience themselves as feeling younger or older than their actual chronological age), it is clear that an individual's mindset has the power to affect the aging process.

Indeed, the mental and physical impact of a person's outlook on aging can be profound. A recent study determined that those who *felt* younger (i.e., those whose attitudes reflected a younger subjective age) had a lower risk of a major depressive episode and a higher chance of flourishing mental health.[2] This same study offered another interesting finding: those who *wanted to be younger than their actual years* had a lower chance of flourishing mental health (and no difference in major depressive episodes). Although the difference may seem subtle, it is an important one to emphasize. In essence, individuals who *felt* younger than their actual age were more likely to have thriving mental health, whereas those who *wished to be* younger were less likely to have thriving mental health. Of course, this research did not investigate all forms of depression, yet it does offer reassurance that an optimistic, vibrant outlook has the power to positively affect certain areas of mental health. Given that so many aging issues are beyond an individual's control, it's comforting to know that one's attitude can help make a positive difference during the aging process.

So as you move forward, remember that a positive, buoyant outlook may reduce your risk for major depression and benefit your overall mental health. Now that's something to smile about. There are many things in life we *can't* change, but it's a powerful truth that our attitude isn't one of them.

Another dose of positivity might be helpful before moving on. Although research indicates that genetics certainly contribute to depression, certain strategies and attitudes have been found to minimize (or even override) a genetic tendency or "set point" for depression. Evidence reflects that approximately 50 percent of an individual's enduring level of joy or subjective well-being (often referred to in research as "happiness") is the result of a genetic set point. Forty percent of an individual's level of joy is the result of intentional activities (behaviors and thought patterns). Amazingly, only 10 percent of an individual's joy level can be attributed to life circumstances. When it comes to finances, research shows that money improves well-being only up to a certain point; once basic needs are met, a greater level of financial resources does not tend to increase happiness.

The beauty of the research findings lies in this key point: an individual's genetic set point for joy can actually be shifted by engaging in positive behaviors and thought processes.[3] So while a person may be born with genetic factors that make it a little easier to be gloomy than joyful, certain strategies can help increase the individual's level of joy.

Wisdom Tip 17: Cultivate a Positive Mindset.

Your daily mindset really matters. Strive to view joy as an internal state that always exists, even if a gray cloud of depression might obscure the joy now and again. Remember that creating joy in your life is a process—a *journey*. You don't "find" joy, you create joy by being mindful of your power to choose optimism over negativity.

You can create joy in simple ways, such as slowing down to notice and enjoy life's daily activities. By using the simple ideas outlined in the upcoming list, "Ten Tips for Easing Depression by Supporting a Positive Mindset"—choosing those that work for you and creating ideas of your own—you will have tools that help you remain more joyful throughout your days. Although these tips won't necessarily "cure" depression, they certainly can help you create a more joyful baseline that will support positive changes.

For those who struggle with chronic depression or other mental health concerns, these simple tips may work well in conjunction with psychotherapy and necessary pharmaceuticals. It's important to stress that such tips are not a "cure" for clinical depression. For those who want to nurture a more generally joyful outlook, continued use of the outlined tips will create truly positive results.

As with any change you want to make, practice is key. The more you practice the tips, the more they will become a natural part of your daily way of being. *Take care to not judge yourself if old patterns try to take hold; just smile and continue to move forward with positivity.*

Ten Tips for Easing Depression by Supporting a Positive Mindset

1. Cultivate a joyful attitude by consciously focusing on the positive in life. If you find yourself fixated on something negative, simply turn to a positive thought or image.
2. Create a positive mantra or two and repeat it as often as you like. Your mantra might be an uplifting blend of thoughts, such as "I am loved. I am truly blessed. I am healthy. I have a new day ahead of me to play and explore."
3. Practice joyful behaviors, such as smiling, dancing, and singing out loud.
4. Consciously "let go" of minor annoyances; release the negative energy.
5. Connect with supportive friends and family as often as possible.
6. Exercise regularly to improve your outlook. Even a quick, fifteen-minute walk can boost your mood by increasing feel-good neurochemicals in your brain.
7. Practice acts of kindness, whether at home, work, or by volunteering.
8. Strive to enjoy the moment as you avoid focusing on the past or overthinking.
9. Practice forgiving life's hurts while also setting firm, kind boundaries for the future.
10. Connect to your sense of spirituality (whether through meditation, organized religion, walks in nature, or other means).

Major depression—which is different from the normal, occasional sense of feeling sad, "blue," or "down in the dumps"—is one of the most common mental health issues. Sometimes referred to as clinical depression, major depression is not to be taken lightly and generally requires professional attention. Depending upon the individual, those suffering from major depression can suffer mild, moderate, or severe impairments in daily life activities. A major depressive disorder is generally diagnosed when a change in functioning occurs during a minimum of a two-week period that involves depressed mood or loss of interest or pleasure; this diagnosis also requires that at least four additional specific symptoms be present during this two-week period. These specific symptoms often include: difficulty concentrating, problems with sleeping or eating properly, irritability, fatigue or loss of energy nearly every day, frequent crying, suicide attempts or recurrent thoughts of death or suicide, and ongoing feelings of worthlessness or inappropriate guilt.

Although depression can occur at any time in life, the National Institute of Mental Health (NIMH) notes that the rate of major depressive episodes is highest among adults between ages 18 and 25. The prevalence is nearly twice as high for adult females (8.5 percent) when compared to adult males (4.8 percent). In the most recent year studied, the NIMH estimated that nearly 7 percent of adults suffered from at least one episode of major depression.[4] It's important to remember that these figures represent only those who have been identified as a result of seeking treatment, thus not reflecting those who suffer in silence.

Whether or not you or a loved one suffers from major depression or other depressive disorders, it is important to be as informed as possible. Although depression is fairly common in older women, and older adults in general, depression is *not* a normal part of the aging process. Depression may present itself differently in later adulthood. Whereas younger adults tend to display affective signs of depression, older adults are more likely to exhibit loss of interest, somatic complaints, and cognitive changes. Older adults may also have reduced awareness of the signs of depression, and thus are less likely to disclose feelings of depression. Of course, stressful circumstances and events can trigger depression, thus making later adulthood (which is often filled with stressors) a time to be particularly watchful for signs of depression. Depression can be activated by stressors, such as the death of loved ones, changes in marital status, the diagnosis of a health condition, and hospitalization. Given that serious medical conditions often arise in middle and older adulthood, it's also important to realize that depression can co-occur with health problems such as stroke, cancer, heart disease, diabetes, Parkinson's disease, and fibromyalgia.

Some symptoms of depression (e.g., confusion, concentration difficulties, impaired executive functioning, and changes in memory) may be confused with early stages of certain brain disorders like Alzheimer's disease. Such conditions, sometimes referred to as depressive pseudodementia, respond well when the underlying depression is properly diagnosed and treated. It is also important to note that certain medications prescribed for medical conditions may actually *contribute* to depression. As well, older adults who suffered from depression in younger years are more at risk for developing depression than those who did not suffer from depression earlier in life.[5] Given the variety of changes that occur in different forms and situations during the later years of life, it is clearly important to be aware of and watchful for symptoms of depression.

If you are suffering from depression, reach out for treatment right away. To ensure that you receive a proper diagnosis, consult your physician to obtain a thorough medical evaluation, including laboratory tests. Make certain that a treatment plan for depression includes psychological support and any appropriate medications.

Remember these important truths: If you suffer from depression, it is not your fault. You need not feel ashamed or embarrassed. Depression is something to be faced—not hidden and suffered in silence. If depression is affecting your life, reach out for appropriate support immediately. You *deserve* proper care and attention.

Anxiety and Aging

Given our busy, often unsettling world, it's possible that you are one of the millions of women who suffer from an anxiety disorder. If you keep an anxiolytic in your purse, desk drawer, or medicine cabinet, you are not unusual. Many women are highly attached to their anti-anxiety medications and fear going out into the world (or handling daily home events) without their "anxiety meds." According to the NIMH, nearly 20 percent of the American adult population suffered from an anxiety disorder in the last year studied. Women (with an anxiety disorder prevalence rate of 23.4 percent) were far more likely to suffer from an anxiety disorder than males (14.3 percent). It is estimated that nearly one-third of American adults will suffer from an anxiety disorder at some point in their lives.[6] As with many such statistics, reported data often underestimate the actual figures, for many Americans do not reach out for mental health support.

So if anxiety feels like a "normal" part of your life, trust that you are not alone. If you are suffering from social anxiety disorder, panic disorder, or generalized anxiety disorder (GAD), you are in the company of millions of women (and men). The following statistics from the Anxiety and Depression Association of America are striking and may help reduce some of the anxiety you may have about having anxiety issues.[7]

- Although anxiety disorders are the most common mental health disorder in the United States, less than 37 percent of those affected by anxiety disorders receive treatment.
- Almost half of individuals diagnosed with depression *also* receive a diagnosis for an anxiety disorder.
- Women are twice as likely as men to suffer from panic disorder.
- Women are twice as likely as men to suffer from generalized anxiety disorder.

- Approximately 36 percent of those who suffer from social anxiety disorder reported experiencing symptoms for at least ten years before seeking help.

As with many mental health issues, an individual may be predisposed to an anxiety disorder due to a combination of factors that include genetic factors, personal history, brain chemistry, and personality. If you are suffering from an anxiety disorder, it's important to seek professional assistance. Remember, mental health issues like anxiety are *not* your fault. You are not defective, too sensitive, or "broken"; you simply have a mental health concern that needs appropriate attention.

With these sobering facts and reassurances in mind, it's time to turn to what you *can* do on a daily basis to reduce any anxiety you might have. First, it's important to know that not all anxiety is "bad." Indeed, anxiety can be a powerful tool in life; it is one of the ways the body and mind handle fear. Anxiety can arise as a powerful "gut force" that lets you know something is off or not right for you. As well, a low level of anxiety (sometimes termed *optimal anxiety*) can be helpful in getting you motivated to get up in the morning, handle mundane tasks, and function at your optimal level. Higher levels of anxiety and chronic anxiety, however, can actually interfere with daily life and have a negative impact on your physical and psychological well-being.

Whether you have a full-blown anxiety disorder or suffer from mild anxiety now and again, the following outlined tips will help you stay calmer and more at ease during life's challenging periods. As one wise and beautiful woman in her mid-fifties recently noted, "Transition times can be ridden with anxiety . . . It's best to be prepared." And so, take a deep breath. Smile with a bit of joy, and imagine yourself using these tips—and those you create on your own—to reduce anxiety in your life. With a few calming tools in your pocket, you'll be better prepared for whatever life brings.

Wisdom Tip 18: Reduce Anxiety with Tender Care.

You can learn to notice and ease your anxiety as it begins to arise. By "getting ahead" of your anxiety, you can feel more at ease in life. Indeed, when you are more aware of your anxiety, you will be better able to face and manage it instead of feeling as if it's controlling you.

Nine Tips for Anxiety Management

1. Learn to breathe deeply and fully. By focusing on your breath as you count to four with each slow inhalation and doing the same for each slow exhalation, you are slowing down your body's alarm system. Simply put, conscious breathing techniques of this sort bring your calming parasympathetic nervous system online.

2. Notice when anxiety begins to arise. Rather than "pretending it's not there," give yourself a time-out to tend to breathing and self-soothing.

3. Stabilize and soothe yourself when anxiety begins to percolate. You can do this by sitting on the ground, gently tossing a squishy ball from one hand to another, taking a shower, placing your flat hands on a cool wall, or holding a favorite soothing item (e.g., cool, smooth rocks).

4. Take care to notice what triggers your anxiety. When possible, avoid the situations or people that are triggers until you are better able to manage your anxiety.

5. Notice if a trigger is actually a signal that a situation or individual is harmful to you. If this is the case, consider the message within your anxiety; you may need to set firm boundaries or remove yourself from the situation entirely.

6. Create a personalized "calming kit" to carry with you. Your kit may contain lavender oil or another essential oil that you find calming. You may want to include a soothing photo, calming hand lotion, "worry beads," or a comforting mint.

7. Practice daily anxiety-reducing activities, such as meditating, journaling, yoga, and prayer.

8. Strive to surround yourself with music and sounds that are *soothing* rather than stimulating.

9. Exercise in ways that feel calming and positive for you. Whether you take a walk in a city park, run on a treadmill, or take a tai chi class, regular exercise can reduce anxiety.

Notice what works for you in the anxiety-reduction realm. Do more of what makes you feel calmer, and do less of what makes you feel anxious or irritated. Seek support for your anxiety issues, whether from a trusted friend, individual psychotherapy, or group therapy. Remember, too, to consult your primary care health provider for a thorough evaluation, including lab tests. If your physician prescribes anti-anxiety medication, consider it as one important element in your anxiety-reduction toolkit. As always, certain strategies and tools are not a replacement for necessary attention from health care providers, yet they can work beautifully with an on-target professional treatment plan.

The Connection between Subjective Age and Your Beautiful Brain

If the above paragraphs made you feel a little concerned, remember that you do have a powerful ability to affect certain aspects of your aging process. Indeed, an upbeat, vibrant outlook may actually keep your brain and cognitive abilities on the younger side.

On a physiological level, recent research in the field of neuroscience found that subjective age (the age you *feel*) is associated with the process of brain aging.[8] Researchers utilized data obtained from elderly participants' subjective age surveys as well as magnetic resonance imaging (MRI) brain scans; this dual-pronged approach makes their research results even more compelling. The study findings revealed that individuals who perceived themselves as younger than their actual age showed both larger gray matter volume and younger predicated brain age. This significant research suggests that an individual's subjective age is closely related to both physiological brain aging and neurocognitive health in later life.

What does this mean to you? If you *feel* younger than your actual age, your brain and mental functioning may benefit in the long run. So the next time you look in the mirror, you might want to remind yourself (and your beautiful brain) that you are a most extraordinary, vibrant, glass-three-quarters-full, amazing woman. Jaded, worn, and pessimistic? *Never!* Spirited, powerful, and optimistic? *Certainly!*

Wisdom Tip 19: Keep Your Brain Healthy and Vibrant.

As you are learning, you can cultivate a positive mindset and vibrant brain. The following tips (which will support your healthful journey in chapter 3) will help you on your way.

Five Tips to Keep Your Brain Healthy and Vibrant

1. Focus daily on feeling vibrant; keep your age-positive mindset in gear.
2. Be proactive in reducing stress-inducing factors in your life.
3. Try *new* activities, such as learning foreign languages, taking up a new form of exercise, novel crossword puzzles, innovative word games, or engaging in new creative interests like painting or music.
4. Connect with loving, supportive friends and family as often as possible.
5. Eat healthfully, get seven to eight hours of uninterrupted sleep per night, and drink plenty of fresh water.

Whether you are in your fifties, sixties, or beyond, trust that you can make positive changes that will affect your daily life. By keeping your brain as healthy and vibrant as possible, you have the power to affect your aging process. It's never too late to create positive attitudes and habits that will help you love yourself and your amazing life.

The Family and Friendship Connection

Everyone feels lonely now and again. When it comes to the later years of life, loneliness can certainly impact both physical and mental health. Sadly, those who suffer from loneliness often silently suffer alone. In fact, it's sometimes difficult to ferret out the difference between being lonely and being alone.

Loneliness can stem from feelings of being ignored, disconnected, isolated, or marginalized. An individual can feel lonely in a crowded room, busy household, or jam-packed movie theatre. Being alone, however, is not necessarily connected to feeling lonely. Certain individuals thrive when they have a great deal of alone time; such people may rarely feel lonely as a result of their natural, solitary proclivities. Other individuals may have a high need for connection with others; such people often thrive when in the midst of social events, busy work environments, and family activities.

Yet our society is moving in a direction that leaves many people feeling increasingly lonely and often disenfranchised. Given the mobile nature of our population, it's common for family and friends to move hundreds or thousands of miles away. It's now increasingly rare to find several generations of family members living in one household. The comfort of having one's child, mother, and other immediate family in one home (or at least the same town) is increasingly a thing of the past. As messy and busy as such households may have been, they did offer a sense of connection and protection against the rigors of life. Indeed, they offered a form of social insurance—a sense that someone would be close to help those in need. Come what may, be it financial issues or the forces of old age, someone would be there to love and care for those less fortunate or in need.

The more mature years of life often bring newfound loneliness. When children move away to begin their adult lives, a once-busy home can feel terribly empty and lonely. Although some find the newfound quiet and space delightful, many women feel a sense of emptiness and purposeless, particularly if their lives were previously highly oriented toward their children and family life. In addition, many working women find connection through their employment environments. As work relationships often fade after retirement, a sense of disconnection and loneliness can arise. When these issues are coupled with the sense of disorientation and purposelessness, loneliness can become a rather menacing beast. To make matters worse, many lonely people are afraid of telling others that they are lonely. Worried that they will be pitied, rejected, or burdensome, those who feel lonely often fear reaching out for the very thing they need—connection to others who care about them.

Creative Connections: Think Outside the Box

There is no replacement for physical proximity and in-person connection, yet technology does give us options. One lovely woman told me of the joy she finds in staying connected to her friends through an app on her cell phone that allows for video sharing of the daily ins and outs of life. By taking videos of the little bits and pieces of life that are so common to friends (but often missed due to busy lives), friends can stay connected by watching the videos in real time or whenever schedules allow. A non-religious member of my weekly women's group shared that she has found tremendous support by attending a "spiritual center" that offers classes and a wide array of opportunities for connection. Many women I know have formed long-lasting friendships through social clubs, hobby groups, and health-oriented forums. Others have found friend-ship connections through online services that allow meeting those with similar interests. Although technology has, in some ways, created distance between humans, it can also be harnessed to foster connections.

As with other issues, I entreat you not to suffer in silence. If you are feeling lonely or isolated, trust that there are thousands of people—likely within a mere few miles of you—who feel the same. You are not unworthy or unwanted if you are lonely; you are sim-ply *feeling* lonely. You can do something about this. You can reach out for support and connection.

Wisdom Tip 20: Reach Out to Avoid Feeling Lonely.

You are so lovable. Remember that truth. If you are feeling isolated or lonely, the following tips may be very helpful to you.

Eight Tips to Reduce Loneliness

1. In an open, non-blaming way, reach out to friends and family to let them know you feel lonely. Although you may feel uncomfortable doing this, it's an important first step.

2. Openly and honestly let others know what you need, such as more in-person time at home, regular phone calls, or social outings. Be as specific as possible.

3. If you don't have loved ones to support you (and even if you do), reach out for group therapy, individual therapy, or other trusted sources of support.

4. Get outside! Whether you take a walk, go to the store, or sit in the park, use time outside to engage with others, even if only to smile and chat.

5. Join social clubs. Follow your interests (or engage in new interests!) by joining clubs that promote connection.

From hiking groups to art and gardening clubs, seek out stimulating activities.

6. Volunteering can be a tremendous way to meet others as you give back to your community. Many communities have volunteer centers that can help you find the right fit.

7. Use technology to your benefit. Search online for local groups, apps, and organizations that will support connection to new friends and old friends alike.

8. Welcome others into your world. As it feels appropriate to you, consider holding small group events with friends in your home. From reading clubs to small potluck gatherings, invite others to share your time and space.

Well done! You may now know your strengths and your frailties quite a bit better. You may now understand that your weaknesses are nothing more than places that give you the opportunity to grow. No matter your age—or maybe *because* of your age—you can now utilize your increased awareness to create positive, joyful changes in your life. You are now many steps closer to enjoying your amazing self and the future that life holds for you. As you love yourself more and more from the inside out—as you engage in age-positive thoughts and behaviors—the days and years that come will grow increasingly inviting to you.

Thank you for having the courage to venture into this next phase of your life with optimism, courage, and strength. Thank for having the bravery to spread your amazing, powerful wings. Thank you, too, for being part of the positive change this world so dearly needs.

CHAPTER 3

Appreciating and Caring for Your Beautiful, Maturing Body

*T*his chapter is a tremendous opportunity to get to know your body and become invested in caring for the physical aspects of your being. From perimenopause and sexuality to the latest anti-aging treatments and research, this chapter will explore some of the most common physical and health issues that affect maturing women. Your journey into this realm will be further supported with helpful insights and effective tools.

This will be a very personal chapter, and I encourage you to use it as a foundation to truly honor and care for your overall physical being. I want to take you beyond the details of customary aging-related medical and health information. My goal is to support you in creating a greater awareness that will lead you to understanding, normalizing, and honoring your experiences. Ultimately, I want you to feel empowered to create a terrific relationship with your beautiful, maturing body in a way that is perfect and right for you. I'll be getting very personal and intimate for a key reason: it's important to break through the barriers that have held women in fear, embarrassment, and shame of their own beautiful bodies. Whatever your size or shape may be—whether the years have been kind or not-so-gentle to your physical being—now is the time for you to appreciate and care for the amazing body that has brought you through life thus far.

To this end, I feel it's only right that I share a very personal memory with you. How can I ask you to stand in your skin with pride and vulnerability if I am not willing to do the same with you? And so I'll share a snippet of a certain "coming of age" moment with you. There came a day that my first husband told me in obnoxious terms that he didn't like my breasts any longer. In essence, he apparently expected my breasts to remain as youthful as they were when we'd met in my early twenties. I remember my shock at hearing his words, for my breasts were beautiful to me; they were part of my entire being. They were the breasts that had known teenage bras, prom dresses, and my wedding gown. They were the breasts that had offered nourishment to our two sons. They were the breasts—*my* breasts—that had loved and been loved. My breasts were part of my being.

I recall standing in my bedroom, stupefied by his disparaging comments for a moment or two. Then, with hot tears in my eyes, shame moved in. Not too long after, I felt my anger begin to rise. I remember capturing a glimpse of my body in the mirror and turning to say, "Perfect or imperfect, my breasts are part of the skin that I live within. It hurts deeply that you would dissect me—*your wife and the mother of your children*—in such a way." His toxic words loitered inside me, despite my efforts to shoo them away. I realized with dismay that I now saw my body through the lens of his tainted perspective. "*What can I do about this?*" I asked myself. "*I want to love my body again!*"

How ridiculous it is to expect a body—to even *want* a body—to not reflect the passage of time and the lovely wear marks of life's journey. Although it was not his intention to do so, my first husband unwittingly gave me a few tremendous gifts through his noxious comments. One gift came in my learning that such an attitude was simply unacceptable to me. My psyche cringed at the thought of being judged in such a way. My body recoiled at the feeling of being so disrespected. I knew that I never wanted to know that feeling again. A second blessing was my coming to deeply understand the importance of being with those who love us with all our lovely characteristics *and* imperfections. A third gift came in the form of my feeling empowered to embrace my body as it was or (if *I* so desired) pursue a cosmetic remedy. As a powerful bonus, I realized that such judgmental attitudes should be unacceptable to all of us—both women and men. So if you detect a hint of ferocity in my tone, I hope you join me in being ferocious for the right reasons. If anyone—even yourself—demeans you for your physical characteristics, feel free to gently and respectfully set them straight. Your body is your home. It is the temple of your psyche and your soul. Your body is a gift and treasure; it is part of you.

Now, as we venture forward together, you know a little more about me. I hope my sharing helps you know a little more about yourself too. After all, we are quite similar as women. We have far more in common than what we don't. We have the bodies of women. We have the souls of women. Our spirits are united by womanhood. It is my goal to focus on our commonalities while also allowing every woman to create a space that supports her individuality. As you read, let your gut instinct guide you toward the path that is right for you. There is no right or wrong way to age beautifully; there is only the way that is right and true for you. What is most important (and I will stress this throughout these pages) is that you feel beautiful within your own skin. Whatever you choose to do or not do is your decision. No choice is a "bad" one as long as it is healthy for you.

I want you to look in the mirror and find yourself beautiful. I want you to do (or not do) whatever allows you to feel joyful and at ease in your own skin. As you consider certain tips, regimens, and procedures to make yourself feel more radiant, be sure to follow your heart. If, however, you find yourself adjusting who you are—physically or otherwise—to please someone else, take pause. Notice what it is that brings *you* joy. And then, with a dose of wisdom and a knowing smile, follow what feels right for you—powerful, amazing, beautiful you. Our goals then, as women, might be these: to not judge ourselves or others as we make choices to engage in practices that allow us to look and feel our best, to shirk off shame and embarrassment as we explore this new frontier with grace, and to embrace ourselves and each other in the journey of thriving and aging joyfully.

Recommended Health Care Visits for the Maturing Woman

Many women are very adept when it comes to taking care of others, yet they don't do very well at caring for themselves. When it comes to your health care and medical needs as you age, it's important to prioritize yourself. Remember, your body has served you well for decades. When you come from a place of gratitude for your physical being, proper health care becomes a joy and a privilege. Although health care organizations and physicians don't always agree on the timing and nature of the most vital medical screenings for maturing women, the outline below will give you a great start. For those with medical conditions such as heart disease or diabetes, it's important to consult your primary care physician as certain screenings may be required more frequently, based upon your situation and general health. However, even if you feel like you are in top physical shape, routine health screenings are vital—they may even save your life.

Unfortunately, our health care system is often "sick care" rather than care designed to promote and preserve overall health and wellness. Although we want to believe that our health care providers are focused on amplifying and supporting our health, they are frequently bogged down in attending to illnesses. Yet people are hungry for wellness; they want to live healthy lifestyles that foster greater energy and positive habits that will keep them out of doctor's offices and hospital rooms. If you are one of the many women craving true health care rather than sick care, here's a tip: You will need to become your own health care advocate. You will need to adjust your role from unaware patient to that of a focused and mindful wellness-oriented client.

For starters, get used to the idea of arming yourself with an arsenal of current and historical health data. When you make a visit to your health care provider, have a written outline of your concerns. You'll also want to have a detailed outline of your personal medical history from birth forward, as well as an outline of your family history. In fact, there's no time like the present to ask your parents and close relatives for details on family history. Ask yourself this important question: Who do I need to interview before they die? Although this might be a sensitive area for some, it's important to obtain this information for your own health.

When you interview family members, ask for relevant details, including each parent's health concerns (e.g., history of cancer, blood pressure issues, cardiac issues, stroke, diabetes, etc.). When possible, obtain age of onset and timeframes for each health condition, actions taken to address the health condition, age at time of surgeries or medical events, mental health issues, and medications used. When you are armed with your important personal medical history, you'll be in a better position to advocate for yourself, and your health care provider will be able to give you the personalized attention you deserve. If the idea of being your own health and wellness advocate is new or frightening for you, trust that the wisdom tips outlined in this chapter will help you become a savvier wellness-oriented client.

When writing this book, I consulted with an excellent physician on healthcare topics. She said to me, "It's important to get the most out of your visits to your doctor's office. In truth, the patient has an agenda, the doctor has an agenda, and the system has an agenda. The ideal patient is one who is a self-advocate. This shows respect for the self, the physician, and the physician's time. It's wonderful to work with those who are involved in their own care—those who truly want to be healthy and are invested in their own health.

"People often think that something that happened to them a long time ago doesn't matter anymore. They forget to report tonsillectomies, appendectomies, and gallbladder surgeries—all of which are important for a physician to know about. Patients need to be self-informed; they need to be able to tell their doctor if they were products of a normal vaginal delivery, if they had a twin that died, and when they were vaccinated. As a physician, it's important for me to know if a patient has a first degree relative with colon cancer, prostate cancer, breast cancer, heart disease, etc.—all of these facts are vital to giving the patient appropriate care. Some people don't realize how important it is for me to know certain details, such as when they started smoking, when they stopped smoking, or how many alcoholic beverages they drink a day. It's so helpful when a patient can tell me when their cholesterol was last checked and what the numbers were. All of this is relevant and necessary when it comes to treating a patient.

"It's important for women—for all patients—to know that a physician needs a thorough outline of a patient's personal and family health history. When a doctor doesn't have a patient's relevant medical history, recommendations are generally based on population-based data. That's how evidence-based medicine works. Yet, patients can be far better served when they provide details on personal genetic makeup, current state of health, and a full health history. This makes the process much more efficient and individualized. As a doctor, I want to make recommendations based on the individual in front of me, not on general, population-based data. And there's a difference between health-span and lifespan. A patient's lifespan can be increased with medical care, but it's actually an individual's health-span that is most important. A long life without good health isn't the ideal. The ultimate goal is to have a truly healthy lifespan."

Let this physician's honest, straightforward guidance support you in becoming an empowered self-advocate. An informed and aware wellness-oriented client is far more likely to obtain personalized, appropriate care. Through this lens, we can move away from sick care and into the arena of health and wellness care.

With the preceding information in mind, it's important to emphasize that health care screening guidelines are population-based and may not be ideal for you as an individual. Utilize these guidelines as educational points rather than what is necessarily *ideal* for you. As you step into the role of an empowered health and wellness self-advocate, you will be able to partner with your physician to determine what is appropriate for you based on your unique needs and overall health history. The current basic recommended guidelines—generally outlined for those in their fifties and sixties, unless otherwise noted—are described in alphabetical order below. Those in other age groups or with existing medical concerns should refer to their primary care providers for specific recommendations.[1, 2]

- *Blood Pressure Screening*—Yearly. More frequent screenings may be necessary if your readings are above the recommended numbers or if you have other health concerns, such as diabetes, kidney problems, or heart disease. Consult your health care provider to determine what is best for you.
- *Breast Exam*—Monthly. Make it a practice to touch your own body—including your beautiful breasts. Your health care provider may also perform a breast examination as part of your routine care. Always contact your health care provider promptly if you notice any changes in your breasts or other areas of your body.

- *Cholesterol Screening*—Yearly. Cholesterol screenings generally begin between ages forty and forty-five and are recommended every five years after the first check. Women in their forties, fifties, sixties, and beyond should be screened at least every five years if they are in good health. Those who have medical conditions such as diabetes, heart disease, kidney problems, and high cholesterol may require more frequent screening. Consult your health care provider to determine the screening frequency that is optimal for you.
- *Colorectal Cancer Screening*—Yearly to every ten years, depending on the test. For healthy individuals, screening generally begins at age fifty. Tests and testing frequency may may vary depending on your history and risk factors. The types of tests available and the related screening intervals are as follows:
  - » Stool-based test (fecal occult blood)—Yearly.
  - » Fecal immunochemical test (FIT)—Yearly.
  - » Stool DNA test—Every three years.
  - » Flexible sigmoidoscopy—Every five years.
  - » Double-contrast barium enema—Every five years.
  - » CT colonography (virtual colonoscopy)—Every five years.
  - » Colonoscopy—Every ten years.
- *Dental Exam*—Every six months or yearly. Depending on your dentist's recommendations, a dental cleaning and exam is recommended at six-month or yearly intervals.
- *Diabetes Screening*—Every three years. If you are in good health, it is recommended that you be screened for diabetes every three years if over age forty-four. Earlier or more frequent screening is often recommended for those who are overweight or have other diabetes risk factors. Those with a family history of coronary artery disease or stroke need to take extra care, as diabetes is increasingly correlated as a contributor to these conditions. People

are frequently diagnosed with diabetes *years* after having initially developed it.

Due to increased risk for developing diabetes, Asian Americans with a BMI (body mass index) greater than twenty-three should be screened as recommended by their health care provider. Consult your primary health care provider to determine what is optimal for you.

- *Eye Exam*—Every one to four years. From age forty to fifty-four, an eye exam is recommended every two to four years. From age fifty-five to sixty-four, an eye exam is recommended every one to three years. For those age sixty-five and older, an eye exam is recommended every one to two years. For those with diabetes, a yearly eye exam is recommended. As well, if you have vision problems or are at risk for vision problems such as glaucoma, more frequent eye examinations may be recommended. Consult your eye care provider for specific recommendations.

- *Hearing Test*—As required. If you experience any symptoms of hearing loss, it is important to consult your health care provider to schedule a hearing test.

  Note: If your care provider recommends hearing aids, take prompt action. Your hearing (your ability to filter noise) will suffer if you delay using recommended hearing aids.

- *Immunizations*—As needed.
  - » Many health care providers recommend a yearly flu shot; consult your health care provider to determine what is best for you.
  - » Ask your health care provider if a pneumonia vaccine is appropriate for you. In general, a pneumococcal vaccine is recommended for those over age sixty-five.
  - » If you didn't have a tetanus-diphtheria and acellular pertussis (Tdap) vaccine as an adolescent, this vaccine is recommended. A tetanus-diphtheria (Td) booster is recommended at ten-year intervals.

> » After age fifty, a shingles or herpes zoster vaccine is recommended.
> » Depending on your medical history and risk factors, other immunizations may be recommended by your health care provider.

- *Lung Cancer Screening*—As needed. An annual lung cancer screening is recommended for those age fifty-five to age eighty who currently smoke (*or* quit smoking within the past fifteen years) AND have a history of smoking thirty packages of cigarettes per year. The recommended type of screening is LDCT (low-dose computed tomography).
- *Mammogram*—As needed. From age fifty to seventy-five, mammograms are generally recommended every one to two years. The frequency depends on personal medical history and risk factors; consult your provider to determine what is best for you.
- *Osteoporosis Screening*—As required. A bone density test (DEXA scan) is recommended for all women over age fifty with fractures. Screening is also recommended for all women under age sixty-five with osteoporosis risk factors. Osteoporosis screening is recommended for *all* women over age sixty-five. Consult your provider to determine what is ideal for you.
- *Pap Smear and Pelvic Exam*—Every three to five years. A Pap smear is recommended every three years. In cases where a Pap smear and HPV (human papilloma virus) test are done together, your provider may recommend testing every five years. Note that a pelvic exam (during which your health care provider feels your ovaries with his or her fingers) is the *only* screening for ovarian cancer. More frequent pelvic exams and related tests may be recommended more frequently, depending upon your history and risk factors.

  Women who have more than one sexual partner are at higher risk for STDs (sexually transmitted diseases) and should be screened for gonorrhea and chlamydia, as well as other STD-related issues. More frequent screening (e.g., every six months) may be recommended for those at higher risk for STDs.

Pap smears are not required for women who have undergone a total hysterectomy (removal of cervix and uterus) and have not been diagnosed with cervical cancer. Most women sixty-five and over may discontinue Pap smears if they have not been diagnosed with cervical cancer or precancer *and* have had three negative Pap smear test results within the past ten years. Consult your primary care provider or gynecologist to determine what is best for you.

- *Physical Exam*—Yearly. A routine physical examination is normally recommended on an annual basis. Each exam generally includes: a blood pressure check; an assessment of height, weight, and BMI; a medication review; an alcohol and tobacco use review; a diet and exercise review; a depression evaluation; and a safety evaluation (domestic violence, use of seat belts, etc.). Routine laboratory tests are often recommended to check cholesterol levels (every five years or as required), blood sugar levels (as required), and other important factors. Those with health concerns may require more frequent examinations and lab tests. Consult your primary health care provider to determine what is optimal for you.
- *Skin Exam*—As needed. It is generally recommended that routine physical exams include skin cancer checks. Those with a weakened immune system and those with a personal or family history of skin cancer often require more frequent exams. Consult your health care provider to determine what is best for you.

The preceding list is a general guide to help you create a plan for optimal self-care. As you embrace the role of being your own health and wellness advocate, remember to invest in accruing and maintaining good records on your health care history as well as your family history. This will allow your health care provider to make personalized screening and wellness recommendations that are ideal for you. Your health care needs are as individual as you are!

Wisdom Tip 21: Make Health Care Appointments as Stress-Free as Possible

Health care examinations and medical tests can be stressful on many levels. Appointments can be time-consuming and disruptive to one's schedule. As well, depending upon the nature of the appointment, a woman may certainly feel vulnerable and embarrassed. Financial concerns can also create additional strain. If you are one of the many women who feels stressed when it comes to your medical appointments, it's important to acknowledge this and let your health care provider know how you are feeling. You don't need to apologize or make excuses; you can simply state that you feel anxious or unsettled. If you do know the sources of your anxiety or discomfort, feel free to let your provider know. Of course, remember to engage in good self-care when at your health care provider's office. You might find it relaxing to listen to gentle music using your headphones, read a book, or take a soothing hobby (such as knitting) with you.

Wisdom Tip 22: Request a Thorough Review of Your Intake Forms.

Ensure that your health care provider reads your intake forms. All too often, a woman takes the time to complete a thorough intake form as she waits for her appointment, only to have the provider rush in unprepared and uninformed. Given the busy nature of many provider's schedules, this is understandable—if unfortunate. As a result, it's important for a woman to ask the provider outright if the intake form has been reviewed. If the forms were not reviewed, ask the provider to review the details. This will save time and help ensure that important information is not overlooked.

Wisdom Tip 23: Appreciate Your Health Care Advocacy Needs.

Health care advocates can be essential in certain situations. Some women find it easy to voice their needs, ask questions, and assert their rights. Others only have difficulty advocating for themselves in certain situations, and some feel uncomfortable speaking up for themselves in general. When it comes to your health, it's important to know if you are a strong self-advocate or if you need support.

If health care appointments are particularly unsettling for you and you tend to meekly defer to opinions and recommendations (even when you don't understand them), ask a friend or family member to attend appointments with you. Until you become more comfortable being your own advocate, you may need to have a caring source of support at your side. Remember that even the strongest, most assertive women may need advocates during times of crisis or ongoing health issues. Asking for support is not a sign of weakness; knowing when to reach out is a sign of wisdom and strength.

Wisdom Tip 24: Create a "Health Care Binder."

Create a "Health Care Binder." As your health care awareness increases, you may find that you have been neglecting vital elements of your own self-care. To reduce stress and maximize efficiency, I recommend creating a "Health Care Binder" to help you monitor your health care needs, medical appointments, medications, and medical history. This binder may also be used to help your significant other or family members stay abreast of your health care issues. You may want to place a copy of the above outline for recommended screenings in the front of this binder as a reminder; make special note of your health care provider's personalized recommendations. You can add a notepad to this binder to help you track health care questions as they arise. The notes you make ahead of time will help you feel more prepared for your health care visits. You will feel more empowered and less stressed when you feel in control of your health care.

Make certain that your binder also contains copies of your long-term health planning forms, such as your Advance Healthcare Directive, Medical Power of Attorney, DNR (do not resuscitate) order, POLST (Physician Orders for Life-Sustaining Treatment), and organ donor forms. As you will note in chapter 5, it's tempting to put off long-term planning due to our fear of the unknown. Yet it is better to be clear and in control of how you want to be treated in the event of a health care emergency. This is an essential aspect of taking charge of your own health care and well-being.

Exercising Joyfully

The single most important thing you can do to prevent and reduce the effects of age-related disease is to MOVE your body. Routine exercise is a must for all age groups; indeed, we often look and feel our best when we make exercise a natural part of each day. As well, given the often increasingly sedentary nature of our more mature years, exercise is particularly vital for maturing adults. The human body is meant to move and engage in a wide variety of tasks every day. Yet unlike our fairly recent ancestors, we frequently spend a great deal of time sitting or engaging in routine, generally stationary tasks.

As one's age increases, even those who are accustomed to being active (going to the gym, taking daily walks, or swimming) may find themselves being resistant to the wear and tear of exercise. Whereas a strained muscle may have formerly taken a few days to heal, the body may now require weeks or months of healing time. Those who favor high-velocity sports may find themselves unable to keep the pace and level of activity they once did, and then—out of sheer frustration—move away from sports that now seem out-of-reach. For those who have always been less inclined to engage in physical activity, the later years of life can lead to nearly permanent couch-potato status. But even for those who have long-shunned physical activity, there is no better time than right now to make positive, health-promoting changes. Whether you take careful steps to adjust your type and level of activity to a "can-do" level or begin an exercise program for the first time, it's important to engage in exercise that feels right—and is right—for you. It's never too late to begin a healthy, balanced exercise program. Of course, always discuss the potential changes with your primary care provider before undertaking a new activity or increasing your activity level.

Sadly, research indicates that approximately 80 percent of adults (and adolescents) in the United States are not exercising enough. Although research has proven that exercise reduces the risk of many chronic diseases, such as coronary heart disease and diabetes, many Americans ignore the healthful benefits of regular exercise. And, in truth, exercise is believed to actually reduce the risk of *all* age-related disease. Exercise has also been proven to help people sleep better, function better mentally, and feel better psychologically. So if you are one of the millions of Americans who find themselves sitting more and exercising less, it's important to take the exercise recommendations seriously. Healthy, joyful living—and healthy, joyful aging—depend on regular exercise. It's a simple, proven truth that no pill or "buy now" button can change. Only you—beautiful you—can make the choice and the effort to exercise.

It might feel great to know that you don't need a great deal of exercise to stay healthy. When it comes to exercise, all you need every week is a mere 150 minutes—this is just a bit longer than your average blockbuster movie. Exercising 150 minutes per week (or just about 22 minutes per day) can keep you physically healthy, looking more vibrant, and feeling more positive. Research indicates that 150–300 minutes per week of moderate-intensity exercise (or 75–150 minutes per week of moderate and vigorous aerobic activity) is necessary for optimal well-being. Given that we often aren't sufficiently active and engaging in muscle-building activities such as frequent manual labor, muscle-strengthening activities are also recommended at least twice per week.[3] Although even 22 minutes per day may sound exhausting if you're unused to exercise, don't worry. Like everything in life, we all need to start somewhere. And starting small—even if it's a 15-minute walk per day—is better than not starting at all.

It's also important to note that four types of exercise—strength, balance, flexibility, and endurance—are generally recommended. If you engage in only one form of exercise, certain areas of your body will not receive the attention they need. For example, a gentle yoga class may be perfect for creating greater balance and flexibility, but it may not provide the necessary strength and endurance components. A bit of time lifting weights and running on a treadmill may be necessary to supplement the stretching and balance provided by gentle yoga. This may sound complex, so it might help to think of it this way:

Our not-too-distant ancestors spent their days engaged in a wide variety of physical activities. From planting gardens and hanging laundry to collecting berries and harvesting grain, their days were naturally filled with activities that kept them strong, flexible, and healthy. Our ancestors ate to fuel their work—not just to eat. They woke at dawn and went to bed at dusk, tired and ready for a good night of sleep. Such lifestyles have been the fiber of human life for millions of years. Yet with the onset of an industrialized society, machines perform the difficult tasks for us. As a result, humans are exercising far less than their bodies and spirits need to stay healthy. We have become largely out of touch with our natural rhythm as people—as women.

Exercise is one way to get back in touch with the amazing body that carries you through life. Let it move. Let it stretch. Let it be strong and beautiful. When possible, add in exercise that requires you to move *consciously*, such as dancing, kick-boxing, or tai chi. In whatever ways work for you, get in touch with activities that get you off the couch, away from the desk, and into a luscious, womanly groove.

Your body and your brain will thank you for engaging in regular exercise. Powerful studies continue to show that brain health benefits from regular exercise. From improved memory function to sharper cognitive abilities, regular exercise shines as one of the most significant anti-aging investments you can make. Aerobic exercise (physical activity that promotes oxygen circulation through the blood) is generally believed to be more beneficial to cognitive health than non-aerobic exercise. Aerobic exercise, which is frequently associated with an increased rate of breathing, can be achieved through brisk walking, running, bicycling, and other "cardio" activities.[4, 5]

Research also shows that regular exercise contributes to greater immune health. Immunosenescence, which is the gradual deterioration of the body's immune system over time, is not necessarily an unavoidable part of the aging process. A healthy lifestyle can certainly affect this process. This is an important point, for when the immune system declines, an individual is more susceptible to infectious diseases and a host of pathological conditions, including cardiovascular disease, Alzheimer's disease, and rheumatoid arthritis.[6] The reduction in physical activity that often comes with aging contributes to immunosenescence. Although exercise can't entirely prevent every age-related decline, regular physical activity can bolster and even protect your all-important immune system.[7]

As well, high levels of exercise also serve to maintain muscle health, thus keeping at bay the deterioration of muscle that occurs with the common age-related increase in sedentary behavior.[8] It makes sense that you will feel better, move better, and stay vibrant-looking if your muscles—which support your very bones—are as strong and healthy as possible.

So, whether or not exercise is "your thing," trust that you can *create* a good relationship with physical activity. The key to maintaining good exercise habits is finding activities that are enjoyable, doable, and appropriate for your body and health. Some enjoy organized exercise activities like group yoga classes, spinning classes, or group hikes. Others prefer solitary exercise in the form of quiet walks, treadmill running, or solo biking. Some delight in natural forms of exercise, such as landscaping tasks, house cleaning, and home maintenance. If you aren't enjoying your current exercise routine, pause to take note of what's not working for you. For example, you may realize that you thrive in a structured group classes or that you prefer unstructured, low-key activities. By taking the time to home in on what feels right for you, you're far more likely to remain engaged in your chosen exercise activities.

For those multi-tasking women who enjoy accomplishing more than one mission at a time, consider how you might weave in your exercise with other items on your to-do list. For example, you can use your walking time to catch up on audio books, podcasts, or serenity time. You might go for a run to the post office, the bank, and then the library. If you're craving girlfriend time, a joint hike can take care of exercise and friendship connection all at once. The goal is to create a joyful relationship with exercise that will naturally keep you coming back for more.

If you are afraid to start an exercise program, know that you are not alone. Some women are afraid to exercise for highly personal reasons. Some are fearful of exercising because their bodies are not accustomed to certain activities. They may feel like "fish out of water" in classes where the exercises and moves seem so natural to others. All too often, we unconsciously create inner stories based on our worries or fears. These negative thought patterns can stop us in our tracks. If you find this happens to you, consider imagining how much fun you might have—how many new experiences you might encounter—by engaging in new routines. From personal experience, I know how unsettling it is to try activities that leave you feeling like a misfit. I am not a born athlete, and whatever athletic prowess I may possess is certainly hard-earned; nature did not bless me with natural athletic abilities. Indeed, stick-to-itiveness, self-compassion, humility, and plenty of laughter have come in handy along the way.

Another common barrier to exercise is weight. Many women who are overweight fear being judged by others; sometimes their fears are imagined, and sometimes they are real. In fact, some women's fears and concerns are exacerbated when thoughtless, judgmental comments and insults are directed at them. Such biased, inappropriate behavior leaves some overweight women feeling stuck between the relative safety of inactivity and the desire to exercise to improve their health. In short, if an overweight woman goes out to exercise, she may suffer verbal abuse or discrimination. Yet if she stays inside where she feels safe, her weight issues may stay the same or worsen. If this resonates with you or someone you care about, it's important to face the issue head-on. Whether you obtain assistance in creating a doable at-home routine or find classes that feel supportive and welcoming, know that you are not alone. As women, it is vital that we support each other and not engage in abusive or discriminatory behavior—whether through negative comments, stares, or ostracizing actions.

It's also important to emphasize that overall fitness is the goal—not weight reduction. Being heavy is not equivalent to being unfit, just as being trim or slight doesn't necessarily make a woman healthy. Indeed, a certain amount of fat is healthy and, depending on your body type, can simply be your natural build. In my experience, many women have a natural weight that feels right to them. Rather than being directed by numbers on a scale, this weight is more a reflection of how one feels in her own skin—a combination of feeling fit physically and psychologically. This place (what I call a woman's "power weight") is not a measurement in pounds or kilos, but a measurement of one's sense of fitness *and* overall well-being.

On a personal level, I thrive when I'm at my ideal power weight. I feel fit, I feel healthy, I feel energetic, I feel clean, and I feel strong. No scale can weigh those powerful feelings for me or for you. Find your healthy power weight and embrace it; make your body—and your life—your own.

Wisdom Tip 25: Get to Know Your Preferred Exercise and Activity Styles.

It's important to understand and honor your personal preferences—from the type of activity and cost to whether you prefer to exercise solo or with others.

First, think outside the box and envision the *types* of exercise that are compelling for you. Do you like adventurous activities like mountain biking, or might you prefer a sedate group dance class? Do you like working out inside, or do you enjoy outdoor activities? Do you prefer structured or unstructured activities?

Second, notice if you feel better exercising in the privacy of your home or if a gym or group facility is appealing. Does combining exercise with social interactions bring you joy?

Third, factor in your overall health. Although the sky's the limit, it's very important to consider exercise programs that both you and your health care provider find appropriate and achievable. And while you can always further your abilities, it's important to select activities that are within your range. You're far more likely to continue with a program that leaves you feeling successful instead of disheartened.

Fourth, consider if you do better at achieving your goals when you feel accountable to someone or something. If so, perhaps you'll thrive with a program that includes motivating factors, such as check-in logs, reward systems, or accountability to friends.

Fifth, look at your finances to ascertain what you can afford. You're more likely to stick with an exercise program that fits your budget.

Your awareness of each of these five key issues will help you investigate a variety of activities and select those that are most appealing, comfortable, and appropriate for you.

Whatever type of activities you select, be firm and specific in your commitments. If you thrive on regular solo activities, carve out routine times for your exercise. If group classes are your thing, make advance plans and put them on your calendar. If you're more likely to exercise with friends at your side, invite buddies to join you. When possible, pay for classes or memberships in advance; this may nudge you to fulfill your exercise commitments, as most of us are more likely to use what we've paid for in advance.

Finally, remember that you are more likely to achieve your goals when you set specific, achievable goals that are supported by micro-goals. (Refer to *Wisdom Tip 15* for a refresher on nine easy-to-follow steps to support your desired changes.)

Wisdom Tip 26: Concentrate on Your Current Abilities.

Focus on what you *can* do, *not* on what you can't do! For example, if the effects of lifelong marathon running have left you unable to run as you once did, strive to focus on what you can do—perhaps jogging, hiking, or taking daily walks. If you focus on the "losses" that come with aging, you may get stuck in a depressive mindset.

For those of you who may just now be getting into shape, it's important to focus on what you *can* do. You don't need to be a downhill skier, soccer player, or aerobics aficionado to get proper exercise. Create opportunities for exercise in novel ways, whether it's vacuuming the carpet (a personal favorite), raking leaves, or taking the stairs instead of the elevator. As long as you are taking active steps toward maintaining a regular exercise routine, you are headed in the right direction!

Wisdom Tip 27: Cultivate an Attitude of Gratitude.

Live with gratitude, stay positive, and don't give up. It takes time to create new exercise habits; it's natural to resist a new regimen or want to leave it behind all together. If feelings like these arise, just notice what's happening and get back on track. Of course, newbies can feel anxious and stressed about the idea of exercising. Fears of "not fitting in" (whether due to weight issues or the "wrong clothing") can also cause stress. All of this is normal, so don't let it get in your way. If doubt and anxiety arise, consciously shift to feeling grateful. Focus on your blessings—the first of which may be that you have a body that is healthy enough to move!

As you move forward to create an exercise routine that feels right to you, remember to celebrate yourself. Allow yourself to be encouraged and motivated by knowing that you have the power of choice; with focus and perseverance, you have the power to create healthy, positive changes in your life. Bit by bit, you have the power to leave unhealthy habits behind you. Your body depends on you and your commitment to optimizing your physical and mental well-being. Way to go! You rock. You are worth taking care of.

Eating Healthfully and Joyfully

When it comes to your diet, it's likely no surprise that *what* you eat and *when* you eat affect your health in incredible ways. Your diet affects everything from your skin, heart, and brain to your sleep and general attitude. Here you are, somewhere in the middle phases of your life, looking at yet another opportunity to infuse yourself with greater well-being. Although some of what is outlined below might seem obvious or rudimentary, it's always worth repeating. As you journey forward, remember that you don't need to make massive changes in your diet. In fact, I urge you to make slow and steady modifications that feel doable and maintainable for you. By adopting changes that feel comfortable and achievable, you'll be able to get off fad diets or "yo-yo" dieting and into a lifelong diet that supports your ongoing health. Here, again, it's important that you focus on what is uniquely right for you. When you find the right fit, your diet will not be a penalty, but a healthy way of life— an ongoing plan of action that supports you.

As always, check with your health care provider before making any changes to your diet. Your health care provider may recommend certain medical tests and laboratory tests to ensure that you are in top form. You may also be able to take advantage of healthy eating classes through your doctor's office, local clinic, or community organizations. Many free online resources (such as the American Heart Association's website) offer sound, easy-to-follow guidelines, tips, and recipes. There are many resources available to help you engage in healthy eating and cooking practices that will serve you well in the coming years. There is no time like today to begin showing yourself greater love by eating healthfully.

Lovely woman, please remember that you do not need to make huge changes to your lifestyle; small, steady changes often lead to the greatest long-term success. When you move forward consciously—making one doable, significant shift at a time—you will find yourself eating and living in more healthy ways. Many change-oriented resolutions fail, not because of the person, but simply due to trying to do everything at once. When expectations are too high and goals are unrealistic, it is all too easy to get deflated. Inside of focusing on achieving radical results, focus on creating new daily life rituals that feel good. As you embrace this mindset—creating healthy rituals in your life that bring you joy—change will come to feel like a good and welcome friend.

Now it's time to ask yourself, "What's your relationship with food?" It's important to start from this foundation. Do you love food? Do you hate food? Are you indifferent to food? Some people are true foodies, and others (like me) are relatively indifferent to food. Whether you eat to live or live to eat (or find yourself somewhere in between), it's important to understand the nature of your relationship with food. If you find yourself in a love-hate relationship with food, you might also desire to create a friendship of sorts with food and your eating habits. The goal, of course, is to have a healthy relationship with food that allows you to eat when you are hungry, refrain from eating when you're not hungry, and generally choose foods that are healthful for your body.

Wisdom Tip 28: Explore Your Relationship with Food.

Does food have power over you? Does your relationship with food control many of your thoughts and activities? If these thoughts sound familiar, you are not alone. We live in a culture that is food-centric; eating is a strong focus in our daily lives. Many people eat in order to ease stress, anxiety, anger, sadness, boredom, and loneliness. As well, we frequently use food to feel loved and comforted as a result of confusing behavioral patterns that many of us learned in childhood. This often unconscious outlook can lead to cycles of obtaining "love" and "comfort" by eating in unhealthy ways—and then dealing with a plague of self-hatred afterward.

Ideally, we want our relationship with food to be a simple, healthy balance of "eating the amount of healthful foods that your body needs while also enjoying what you eat," yet eating often gets "charged" in unhealthy ways. If your relationship with food feels out of whack, you can also journal about your relationship with food as a starting point. As a result of journaling, you may remember certain memories or issues that contribute to an unhealthy relationship with food. You might uncover certain thought processes or patterns that have left you feeling stuck (and even helpless) in managing a healthy weight. To further your progress, you may want to join a healthy eating support group to further a positive relationship with food. Of course, you may also want to seek the support of a psychotherapist who specializes in eating issues.

It takes courage to change patterns that were likely created in childhood, yet trust that you have the ability, the courage, and the power to engage in new, positive behaviors that will support a healthy, active lifestyle for years to come. Again, you may want to refer to *Wisdom Tip 15* for a refresher on nine easy-to-follow steps for empowered change.

As we age, our diet becomes increasingly important. Although a healthy diet is vital throughout life, the natural declines that occur with aging can be mitigated when beneficial eating habits are the norm rather than the exception. Indeed, a healthy diet can reduce your risk for chronic diseases, such as Alzheimer's disease, diabetes, and cardiovascular disease.[9] Whether you are already at your ideal weight or desire to lose weight, it may be comforting to know that—unless an underlying medical issue is affecting your metabolism and general health—you can achieve your optimal weight by taking in no more or less than the number of calories your body needs on a daily basis. Just like a car's gas tank, your body needs a certain amount of fuel depending on its daily journey. Although the average women requires about 2,000 calories per day, your own ideal caloric intake depends on a variety of factors, such as your body size, level of physical activity, and age. It's natural that you may want to eat like you did as a youngster, yet adults generally need fewer calories than those who are still growing. Your body simply needs less fuel as your metabolism slows and your lifestyle becomes less active.

A healthy diet does not need to be expensive, time-consuming, or complex. Indeed, a few key points are all you need to know:

- Eat plenty of fresh fruits and green, leafy vegetables.
- Enjoy plenty of whole grains, nuts, and legumes.
- Eat skinless poultry, fish, and lean meats.
- Keep sugar consumption to a minimum.
- Avoid sugary drinks and high-caffeine energy drinks.
- Drink plenty of water and cleansing beverages, such as herbal teas.
- Select monounsaturated fats (found in foods like nuts, avocados, and olive oil) and polyunsaturated fats (present in foods like walnuts, sunflower seeds, salmon, and safflower oil) when possible. Saturated fats are found in foods like butter, cheese, red meat, and coconut oil. Use oils with less than four grams of saturated fat per tablespoon. Limit saturated fat, partially hydrogenated oil (an artificial *trans* fat), and natural *trans* fats.
- Consume low-fat or fat-free milk products. Your best product choice will depend on health factors such as your

cholesterol level; ask your health care provider what is ideal for you.

- Avoid processed foods, such as salty snack foods and sugary cereals.
- Limit alcoholic beverage consumption to no more than one alcoholic beverage per day (i.e., twelve ounces of beer or one five-ounce glass of wine).

When you shift your mindset to see your diet as part of your whole being—as a way to give your body daily doses of good self-care—eating healthfully becomes a joy rather than a chore. Have faith that you can create a healthy relationship with this truly important aspect of your overall well-being.

Cosmetic Procedures: Botox, Fillers, Skin-Tightening, Liposuction, and More

Cosmetics and other beauty enhancements have been part of womanhood for thousands and thousands of years. From Cleopatra's eyeliner and Roman hair dyes to tribal tattoos and neck elongating, women (and men) have been using products and procedures to change their appearance since ancient times. So given the modern world's innovative technologies and cutting-edge cosmetic products and procedures, it makes sense that many women are lining up to purchase the latest treatments. Whether undertaking innovative surgical procedures to reshape "problematic" body areas or engaging in age-reducing treatments, women around the world are investing in making the most of their physical appearance.

The American Society of Plastic Surgeons' most recent annual statistics indicate that 17.5 million surgical and minimally invasive cosmetic procedures were performed in the United States, which reflects a 2 percent increase over the prior year. Such increases are not a novel trend, but the data also reflects that there has been a nearly 200 percent increase in minimally invasive cosmetic procedures alone within the last two decades.[11]

If you've been wondering—*when is enough really enough?*—that's a great question to be asking yourself. The answer is very personal, indeed. What is excessive for one woman may be perfectly reasonable and ideal for another. When it comes down to it, the decision to undertake any appearance-changing procedure (whether as minor as coloring your hair or as major as a facelift) is your decision alone. Of course, you might want to ask your partner or friends for input and advice, yet when it comes to your body, the ultimate choices are yours. That said, it's important to understand and honor your needs before making appearance-related decisions, for your choices may impact you physically, mentally, emotionally, and financially.

A few questions to ponder may include the following: Am I undertaking the procedure to feel better about myself rather than to please or "feel loved" by another person? Have I investigated the possible risks of the procedure? Are the risks (if any) worth the rewards of having the procedure? As I envision myself in the mirror, both before and after the procedure, do I have realistic expectations of the outcome? Do I have the financial ability to have the procedure without maxing out my credit card or creating additional financial stress in some other way? Am I certain that I am not expecting the procedure to heal a difficult personal issue, such as a bad romantic relationship, ongoing depression, or other such challenge?

If your answers to the preceding questions are "Yes!" then it's likely that you are right on track in making changes that will help you feel and look your best. For those who have tried everything—from weight loss and body toning to expensive topical treatments—medical procedures may provide solutions for regaining or creating a more personally desirable appearance.

As one vibrant woman told me, "I am stepping away from the mere number of my age; a number doesn't capture who I am. When it comes to cosmetic procedures, I see them as self-care and as part of my overall self-love. When I look in the mirror, I see a face that is familiar and lovely to me. I want the woman on the outside to reflect how I feel on the inside. When I go in for a cosmetic treatment, I feel as though I am embracing and expressing part of my femininity. I want to take care of myself, and I want to look the way I want to look. I don't focus on the idea of anti-aging procedures; I focus on using what science and technology offer to help me feel better, and part of feeling better is loving the way I look. It's no secret that everything in life feels much better when we feel good about ourselves. When I see a woman in the mirror looking back at me with delight, I feel great. It's just part of my entire life experience." Indeed, when we feel positive about ourselves—body, mind, and spirit—life simply feels more joyful. Do what feels right for you; let that face in the mirror smile back at you.

If you're one of the millions of women interested in or already engaging in cosmetic surgical and minimally invasive procedures, the following statistics might be interesting to you. The top five minimally invasive procedures in the United States during the last year reported were: botulinum toxin type A (e.g., Botox) at 7.23 million procedures; soft tissue fillers (also called "injectables" or "fillers") at 2.69 million procedures; chemical peels at 1.37 million procedures; laser hair removal at 1.1 million procedures; and microdermabrasion at 740,287 procedures. The top five cosmetic surgical procedures in the United States during the last reported year were: breast augmentation at 300,378 procedures; liposuction at 246,354 procedures; nose reshaping at 218,924 procedures; eyelid surgery at 209,571 procedures; and tummy tuck at 129,753 procedures.

Body sculpting, skin-tightening, and non-invasive fat-related procedures are also on the rise. Problem-area fat cells are being reduced, eliminated, and redistributed through a variety of innovative techniques that include injectable medications, vacuum massage, radio frequency, infrared light, and ultrasound. Showing an increase of 19 percent over the prior year, cellulite treatments are the fastest-growing procedure in this realm.[12]

Some of these increasingly common procedures are relatively affordable, yet others can be extremely expensive. For example, "maintenance procedures" like Botox may be required several times per year; depending on the individual's needs and the provider's fees, the cost can range from several hundred dollars per treatment to well into the thousand-dollar-per-treatment range. And once a woman has become accustomed to ongoing maintenance treatments (whether for lip fillers, Botox, or even hair treatments), it can be difficult to get off the treadmill. Some medical offices have reward programs and other cost-savings events. Whether investigating surgery or non-invasive procedures, many women "shop the market" to survey pricing and obtain detailed information on procedures; this is wise, as the cosmetic industry services world is highly competitive and constantly changing. Take care, however, to compare prices and services carefully. It's important to have good rapport and a sense of trust with your provider. When it comes to your precious body, it's never wise to sacrifice excellent quality and top-notch services in favor of a lower price.

All of the above procedures (and countless more) are available for those who have the desire and financial ability to undertake them. If you are considering new treatments, particularly those that are permanent, invasive, and costly, take the time to do your research. You may wish to first consult with your primary care provider for feedback and personalized recommendations. You might then talk with friends to obtain first-hand referrals. After that, interview several providers to ensure that you are comfortable with the staff, the facility, and the pricing. As with other health and wellness routines in your life, remember to have a list of questions to discuss during your interview process with any provider; you will feel more empowered when you are well-informed.

As the relationship with your cosmetic service provider is important, it's essential to find the right fit. Before scheduling your appointment, ensure that you've addressed pragmatic details such as finances, work schedule, possible side-effects, downtime, medications to avoid or take before your procedures, and (in the case of more intensive treatments) post-surgery care and support.

Full Disclosure—What's Right for You

Some women love talking about their issues—whether discussing plastic surgery rigors or the latest in cosmetics and diet routines. Other women are more private about their personal issues and may even feel as though such discussions are invasive. What feels right to one woman may feel very wrong to another. Whether or not a woman wants to reveal and discuss her personal issues is entirely up to her. When it comes to disclosure of one's personal world, there is no set right or wrong way to be. Simply come to terms with what is right for you and allow yourself to hold true to whatever that is.

Good boundaries are essential when it comes to such issues. It is so important that we as women—and as role models—allow each other to create and maintain our own boundaries in the most respectful of ways. If a woman declines to offer you details on what she "had done," allow her that privacy. If another woman wants to relay every aspect of her liposuction and "nip and tuck" procedures, allow her to do so unless if feels uncomfortable for you. If it does feel uncomfortable, it's your right to gently set boundaries that limit discussions to what feels appropriate.

As well, if you are a more private person and reticent to talk about your own personal regimen, surgeries, and the like, that's your choice. You needn't apologize or feel guilty for wanting privacy. If someone asks you about your personal realm and it feels uncomfortable to you, it's appropriate to unapologetically say, "That's very personal to me. I prefer not to discuss those details." Those with good boundaries will respect your clarity.

As women who want to support each other to be our best selves, it is vital that we consistently remember that we are role models for each other and for those who look to us for guidance. When we treat each other with respect, we are showing each other—and the world at large—that we walk our talk. We breed kindness and respect by acting with kindness and respect.

Through all of this, it's extremely important to be aware of the likes of guilt, shame, and embarrassment. Whether you color your hair to avoid "gray shaming" or feel guilty for getting cosmetic treatments, strive to understand what is causing these feelings. When you "make friends" with your emotions and your own needs, you will move away from taking action based on guilt, shame, or embarrassment. You will, instead, act based on what is right for you. Thus, you might find yourself having your hair colored because you love the radiance of your chosen color, rather than as a response to being terrified of showing your grays. You might also choose to let go of any guilt or embarrassment you have about undertaking certain cosmetic treatments—you'll simply see your chosen procedures as a necessary aspect of creating and maintaining the look you want.

When you are at peace with your aging process, you will relax into your chosen patterns and regimens, whatever they may be. You will then be proud of your choices and feel more joyful and serene. You will be aware of your boundaries and aware of what feels right for you. You won't feel the need to make excuses, hide anything, or reveal any sensitive personal details. You will feel free and at peace as a result of knowing that you make choices that are thoughtful, wise, and right for you. All of this positive energy will then radiate from within you, making you look and feel your best from the inside out.

Your Changing Skin and Hair

Your skin—the largest organ in your body—is exposed to a lifetime of sun, irritant, and toxins. As we mature, the signs of life's vicissitudes become more apparent on our skin—whether by an increase in wrinkles, age spots, spider veins, dryness, and a host of other issues. Your hair, too, may be changing in ways that are bothersome or irritating for you. Factors such as your genetic makeup, lifestyle (diet, smoking habits, stress level, etc.), and environmental factors all have an impact on your maturing skin and hair. Although you can't erase some of the signs of the aging process, this chapter will give you some helpful guidance and tips on how to take care of this vital aspect of your physical being.

To start with, a broad-spectrum sunscreen is your greatest secret weapon for healthy skin. Even if you've been a sun worshipper in the past, it's never too late to form a healthy relationship with sunscreen. Whenever you are outside or otherwise exposed to sunlight (e.g., through car windows), utilize a broadspectrum sunscreen with an SPF (sun protection factor) of thirty or higher. (SPF applies only to UVB rays, not UVA rays; it is UVA rays that damage DNA. Thus, broad-spectrum sunscreens are critical!) It doesn't hurt to apply a good sunscreen every day whether you plan to be outdoors or not. Not only will religious use of a broad-spectrum sunscreen help protect against skin cancer, it can also help fade existing age spots and prevent the formation of new age spots. Remember, *broad-spectrum* sunscreen is key!

Sun and a lifetime of weathering the elements is not the only culprit. When a woman enters menopause, the drop in female hormones frequently results in pronounced changes in both skin and hair. The supporting structure of your skin is made up of collagen and elastin fibers. Elastin keeps your skin tight and *elastic*—capable of bouncing back. Collagen, a protein and the primary component of your body's connective tissue and dermis, gives your skin its firmness. Both collagen and elastin are plentiful in youthful skin. However, environmental factors (e.g., sun exposure) and natural aging play roles in the breakdown and loss of these important fibers. Indeed, the level of collagen in a woman's skin decreases significantly during menopause. The abrupt drop in collagen accounts for the often "overnight" increase in wrinkles, jowls, lax skin, and thinning skin. As skin loses its taut firmness, wrinkles and lines become more prominent. Lips may be thinner and lines may appear around the lip area. The delicate skin under the eyes may be thinner or pouched, and eyelids may droop and appear heavier.

Enlarged pores also become more visible due to the decrease in collagen. Research indicates that a woman loses approximately 30 percent of her skin collagen in the first five years of menopause. Thankfully, the decline slows after this initial five-year period to a more moderate decrease in collagen each year for the subsequent twenty years.[13] As we get older, our body's collagen production decreases while the level of collagen degradation increases; we see the results of these changes in the quality, look, and feel of our skin.

As we age, we also lose subcutaneous fat (the layer of fat that sits below the skin). This layer of fat helps skin look plumper and smoother. As a woman loses more of this fat, her face may appear gaunt, particularly below the eyes, in the cheeks, temples, and chin. A loss in cartilage may result in a woman's nose appearing bonier and a drop in the tip of the nose. Particularly after age sixty, women may begin to experience bone loss, often around the mouth and chin areas; the mouth may appear somewhat puckered as a result.[14] Bone loss also creates larger eye sockets; this creates an increasingly hollow look around the eyes. Although many of these changes begin during a woman's thirties, the cumulative changes may not be visible until much later.

If strange new bumps and spots seem to be taking up residence on your face, neck, and other areas of your body, take heart. As a friend memorably said, "I'm getting more barnacles as I age!" Her description of the little growths and changes that seem to appear out of nowhere on one's skin seems quite appropriate. From the appearance of age spots and moles to lesions and rough skin patches, the changes can be disconcerting. Although both non-invasive and surgical procedures may help with these issues on a cosmetic level, it's important to take skin changes seriously. What might appear to be a benign lesion might be the beginning stages of skin cancer. If a "trouble spot" appears, make an appointment to see your dermatologist or primary care provider immediately; cancer can be best addressed in its early stages.

You may also notice that your skin also doesn't heal as quickly as it once did. Indeed, a mature woman's skin may bruise more easily after menopause due to decreased estrogen levels. Given that hormones are important for healing in general, the decline in hormones associated with menopause affects the mature woman's ability to recover quickly from bruises and other injuries. Along with a drop in hormones, more mature skin tends to heal extra slowly due to a variety of additional reasons, including more delicate blood vessels, thinner skin, and reduced immune function. Many women also experience greater skin sensitivity and increased skin dryness due to hormonal changes and decreased sebum production. Those who suffer from skin issues such as rosacea or eczema may notice an increase in symptoms; such issues are related to the body's increased sensitivity and diminished healing abilities. "Trouble spots" of pink, rough, or scaly skin may also arise. If you notice something abnormal, consult your dermatologist promptly; treatments are often readily available.

Adult acne is another issue that plagues many women as they mature. Although most women hope that they had left any acne issues in the past, perimenopause and menopause can trigger pimples and other types of adult acne such as cysts. Here, again, hormonal changes are often the culprit. The easiest, most cost-effective treatments include topical products that contain salicylic acid and other products targeted for adult skin issues. Treatments for teenage and early adult acne are usually too harsh for the adult female's more dry and sensitive skin. When topical treatments don't remedy the situation, it's important to consult your dermatologist to discuss more serious options. As adult acne is frequently related to the hormone testosterone, your health provider may prescribe anti-androgen medications ("testosterone blockers") such as spironolactone or other hormonal treatments. Your dermatologist can help you ascertain the most effective treatment for your situation.

All of these changes are normal and natural; some may be troubling to you, and others may not be bothersome at all. If you are struggling with some of these changes, write out a list of what is irksome or difficult for you. If you like, discuss your concerns with your friends or family members to gain added insight and support. With your list in hand, reach out to your primary care provider to get the professional assistance and tools that are vital for you.

Wisdom Tip 29: Care for Your Skin with Loving Attention.

Take the care of your skin seriously! By following these easy-to-use tips, your skin will be in top form:

- Regular use of a quality, broad-spectrum SPF 30 (or higher SPF) sunscreen. Reapply every two hours when outside. Consistent sunscreen use is your skin's best defense against aging!
- When outside, give your skin extra protection by wearing a hat and sunglasses. Cover exposed skin with protective clothing.
- Avoid sun exposure between 10:00 a.m. and 3:00 p.m. when UV rays are strongest.
- Make an appointment with your dermatologist for a skin-cancer screening. Exams are even more important as you get older, as your risk for skin cancer increases with age.
- Conduct routine skin self-exams to stay on top of changes in your skin. A dark spot or odd-looking "mole" can be cancerous. If you notice something amiss, contact your health care provider promptly.
- Use fragrance-free moisturizers to reduce dryness and increase skin suppleness.
- Avoid artificial tanning, including sunlamps and tanning beds.

- Drink plenty of water and hydrating liquids such as herbal teas.
- Keep your diet as clean and healthful as possible; limit sugar intake and avoid processed foods. A fresh, plant-based diet will help your skin glow naturally.
- Increase consumption of omega-3 fatty acids; foods with high levels of omega-3 fatty acids include walnuts, chia seeds, salmon, oysters, soybeans, and mackerel.
- Consider using skin care products that contain retinoids (derivatives of vitamin A) or peptides, as these products can increase skin collagen.
- Avoid harsh, drying face cleansers and facial products, as adult skin is more sensitive than younger skin. What may have worked in the past may no longer be beneficial.
- If you have adult acne, use adult-acne products to protect your skin from overdrying.
- If age spots, the dark spots on skin resulting from increased skin pigment (melanin) production, or other cosmetic issues bother you, consult your dermatologist for recommendations. Products containing hydroquinone and kojic acid are effective treatments for age spots. Tretinoin cream, laser therapy, and other treatments can also reduce the appearance of age spots and other irksome skin concerns.

As you age, your hair and scalp may show noticeable changes. A woman's scalp may feel dry and itchy. Her hair may start to thin and loose some of its former luster. Some women notice that the hairline starts to recede. Others notice an overall thinning and loss of hair—sometimes most obvious at the crown of the head or part line. If your hair loss is worrisome, consult a dermatologist as soon as you notice changes. Treatments are available for hair loss, and professional guidance can be extremely helpful in finding the best solution. One common treatment is the use of non-prescription minoxidil (a common medicinal treatment for certain hair loss issues) that is applied to the scalp. Those who benefit from minoxidil usually see results within the first few months of treatment and continue to enjoy benefits as long as the product is used. Other treatments include low-level laser therapy (to stimulate hair follicles to grow new hair) and hair transplants (a surgical option for certain cases).

Of course, hair also begins to turn gray as the body's production of melanin decreases. Depending upon one's genetic makeup, hormones, lifestyle, and environmental factors, hair can begin turning gray in a woman's twenties or thirties. Many women, however, find that their hair is most noticeably gray during their forties and fifties. In rare cases, a woman may not experience substantial graying until she is well into her sixties. If your mother or father went gray early, chances are that you'll follow in their footsteps.

Unwanted facial hair (particularly along the jawline, chin, and upper lip) can also arise as a result of imbalances in testosterone and estrogen levels. Tweezing and waxing these spotty hairs provide a temporary solution. For permanent removal, electrolysis is often the ideal treatment. Professional laser hair removal is an option for some, although light color or gray hair does not generally respond well to laser removal treatments. Your dermatologist can also prescribe a hair-reduction cream if unwanted facial hair is excessive and problematic for you.

It's also important to take a look at shingles, a fairly common—and often painful—skin condition that can develop in one's more mature years. Although shingles (caused by the varicella-zoster virus) most frequently occurs in those over fifty, it can affect any person who has had chickenpox. If you had chickenpox as a child or later in life, the virus remains dormant in your nerve tissue near the spinal cord and brain. The virus can be activated by a variety of factors, such as stress, weakened immune system, chemotherapy, and transplant operations. Many adults have only one encounter with shingles during their lifetime, whereas those with compromised immune systems may suffer several bouts. Shingles generally appears only on one side of the face or torso and presents as a band or patch of raised dots. The first symptoms of shingles are tingling, itching, burning, or shooting pain on one side of the face or torso. A rash also appears in a band or patch of raised, irritated dots. Tiny blisters filled with fluid then form and eventually begin a crusting process as they dry out. During its most uncomfortable stages, shingles pain can range from mild irritation and itching to intensely disruptive pain. It's important to contact your primary care physician immediately, as the duration and intensity of shingles can be reduced by prompt treatment with antiviral medications.

Unfortunately, those who have had shingles may continue to experience severe nerve pain well after the rash has disappeared. Known as postherpetic neuralgia, this condition can be very persistent and distressing. The risk of developing postherpetic neuralgia can be lessened by immediate treatment with antiviral drugs.[14] Fortunately, effective shingles vaccines are now readily available. As the risk of developing shingles increases with age, this vaccine is recommended for all adults age sixty and older. *Even if you've already had shingles, you can have the shingles vaccine.* Your primary care physician can advise you on what is best for your age and general health.[15]

Perimenopause and Menopause: Hot Information and Tips

Shhhhhh! We are entering secret territory here. Seriously? It's time that we talk about the big "change of life" in an open, honest way. When it comes to aging issues, the "change of life" topic has too often been either ignored, secreted, minimized, or over-amplified. Whether exploring perimenopause or menopause, the issues needn't be any more confusing or worrisome than the other changes that come in a woman's life.

Just as every woman experiences the shifts that occur with puberty and beyond in distinctively personal ways, the changes that come later in life will be unique to every woman. Yet as certain commonalities do exist, we will explore both the ordinary (and sometimes extraordinary) permutations of perimenopause and menopause. There's no reason to take a secretive or stand-offish stance when it comes to these issues. They are, after all, just another part of your beautiful journey through life. As resisting and ignoring such issues doesn't help at all, it seems quite wise to openly and joyfully embrace the changes!

For those of you who are happy to be moving past a lifetime of menstrual cycles, pregnancy, and child-rearing, this may be a most beautiful time for you. Indeed, menopause is the official marker of the end of a woman's reproductive years. For those who are ready and wanting to move into a new kind of freedom—body, mind, and spirit—these stages in your life may hold more relief than worry or irritation for you. When we look at perimenopause and menopause as entry points into a new and delicious stage of life, any discomforts may seem entirely more bearable.

Perimenopause is the stage in a woman's life when she is transitioning toward menopause. Although we might wish there were certain "starting" and "ending" dates for this stage—something we might be able to count on—it is generally less predictable than we'd like. The changes can be subtle and gradual for some women, whereas others may experience fairly radical and abrupt shifts. Your family history, such as the age your mother began her changes and the symptoms she experienced, may give you an indication of what's in store for you.

Perimenopause simply means "around or near menopause" and refers to the phase when a woman's body gradually decreases its production of estrogen—the primary female hormone. During a woman's reproductive years, her ovaries (organs that also act as the reproductive glands that store eggs and release them into the fallopian tubes) are hard at work producing the female hormones progesterone and estrogen, as well as the hormone testosterone. Estrogen and progesterone work together to control menstruation in addition to other important physiological functions. For example, estrogen affects the body's cholesterol levels and also the use of calcium. As a woman's ovaries become less active during perimenopause, it is the decrease in the production of estrogen that is the most influential factor. The decline in estrogen levels is not linear, and this results in erratic rises and falls in hormone production. This uneven pattern often leads to a host of irritating symptoms such as vaginal dryness, irregular periods, hot flashes, mood swings, and sleep difficulties.

Toward the end of perimenopause—generally the last one to two years of this stage—the reduction in estrogen production accelerates and a woman may experience menopausal symptoms. Progesterone (sometimes called the "pregnancy hormone" due to its important role in promoting fertility and gestation) is another important female hormone that also begins to decline during perimenopause. The fluctuating shifts in female hormones are a natural and normal—if often uncomfortable—aspect of moving out of one's reproductive years.

Although some women are in perimenopause for only several months, perimenopause usually begins in a woman's forties and often commences eight to ten years before menopause (which lasts around four years). Some women may move into perimenopause as early as their thirties, and a few may not shift into this phase until their early fifties. A woman continues to have her period during perimenopause, although her cycles may become more irregular. Given that she is still releasing eggs, a woman may still become pregnant during her perimenopausal years. She may also have periods without ovulating (without the release of eggs). The perimenopause stage segues into menopause when the ovaries no longer release eggs. Perimenopause officially ends—and meno-pause begins—when a woman has not had her period for twelve months.[16, 17]

As always, it's essential that you consult your primary care provider if you experience symptoms that are unusual or bother-some. Given differences in pain tolerance and sensitivity, what one woman finds manageable or merely a "blip" may be disconcerting to another. As well, some women experience significant and stress-inducing symptoms whereas others may find their symptoms rather subtle and tolerable. It is also important to note that any symptoms can feel much worse when other life stressors are present, such as a difficult romantic relationship, work challenges, or childrearing issues. A woman may experience some or all of the common symptoms listed in the following outline as she begins her transition into menopause. It's always a good idea to consult with your primary care provider if any symptoms are at all concerning to you.

Symptoms commonly experienced in perimenopause include: (listed alphabetically)

- *Fertility changes*: For women who are trying to conceive, a change in fertility may be noticed. For those who do not wish to become pregnant, birth control is recommended until the time that twelve months have passed without a menstrual cycle.
- *Increased PMS symptoms*: Premenstrual symptoms such as irritability, food cravings, and breast tenderness may be more intense at times during perimenopause.
- *Irregular menstrual cycles*: Cycles may become less frequent and irregular; skipped periods are a common occurrence during perimenopause. The flow during periods may be irregular, with some months being heavier or lighter than normal. If the flow of your period is much heavier than normal or if the duration is substantially longer or shorter than normal, promptly contact your primary care provider.

  As well, it's important to contact your health care provider immediately if you experience spotting after your period, blood clots during your period, or bleeding after sex. Although such symptoms may be indicative of readily treatable issues such as fibroids and hormonal fluctuations, it's important to rule out highly serious conditions like cancer.

Symptoms common to both perimenopause and menopause include: (listed alphabetically)

- *Bladder issues:* Bladder control issues like incontinence may arise as a result of a loss of tissue tone and elasticity. Some women experience urinary urgency (the pressing need to urinate more frequently) or stress incontinence (urine leakage when coughing, sneezing, or lifting heavier items). A later section addresses this important topic in greater detail.

- *Bone loss:* As estrogen levels decline, bone loss occurs more rapidly. This increases your risk for osteoporosis, a condition that leads to fragile, more easily broken bones.

- *Cardiac symptoms:* Particularly during hot flashes, some women experience a racing heart. Other cardiac symptoms that may occur during perimenopause and menopause include heart palpitations, dizziness, numbness, and tingling. If you experience new or worrisome heart issues of any nature, it is important to contact your primary care provider to rule out a serious heart condition.

- *Changes in cognition:* The ability to concentrate and focus may diminish at times during perimenopause and menopause. Some women experience an increase in forgetfulness and distractibility. (And, no, in most cases, these changes are *not* due to dementia; they can often be attributed to lack of sleep, increased stress, and hormonal fluctuations.)

- *Cholesterol level changes:* Blood cholesterol levels may be affected by declining estrogen levels. The level of LDL (low-density lipoprotein)—the "bad" cholesterol—may increase and the level of HDL (high-density lipoprotein)—the "good" cholesterol—may decrease. These changes, which are the opposite of what we'd like to have occur, may increase a woman's risk of heart disease.

- *Headaches:* As the ovaries produce less estrogen, some women experience an increase in headaches. Just as with other changes that may arise, it's important to contact your primary care provider if headaches are persistent or worrisome.

- *Hot flashes:* Hot flashes (brief, periodic increases in body temperature) are very common during perimenopause and are the most common reported symptom during menopause. Some women do not experience hot flashes at all. Many, however, experience hot flashes a few times a week, several times per day, or even hourly. Although the nature and intensity of hot flashes will differ for every woman, they generally involve feelings of intense heat or flushing in the face, neck, or chest. Skin reddening, rapid heartbeat, and sweating may also occur. If a great deal of body heat is suddenly lost, the hot flash can result in feeling chilled after the hot flash subsides.

  Although the precise cause of hot flashes isn't known, they are believed to be a result of a decrease in estrogen levels and changes in the hypothalamus (the body's thermostat), which may become more sensitive to slight variations in body temperature during perimenopause and menopause. Women who smoke, have a high BMI (body mass index), and are of African American descent are more likely to have hot flashes.[19] Approximately 75 percent of women experience hot flashes to some degree. A sizeable 80 percent of women experience hot flashes for just two years or less[20]; some women, however, experience hot flashes for up to several years.

- *Loss of energy:* Whether as a result of sleep disruption, hormonal fluctuations, or other factors, some women feel less energetic or depleted during these life changes.

- *Loss of fullness in breasts:* As a result of decreased levels of reproductive hormones, a woman will find that her breasts lose firmness and fullness. This is a normal and natural aspect of the aging process.

- *Mood changes:* The fluctuations in female hormones during menopause may contribute to irritability, mood swings, anxiety, or depression. Given that sleep is frequently disrupted during perimenopause and menopause, mood changes may also be attributable to loss of sleep and the resulting increase in sensitivity.
- *Muscle and joint aches and pains:* Given the fluctuations in female hormone levels, some women experience aching or painful muscles and joints. The level of discomfort experienced can be very mild or highly uncomfortable.
- *Sexuality concerns:* A loss of sex drive may be experienced by some women. Those who have had satisfying sexual intimacy patterns in the past may not notice a change. Some women experience increased libido as a result of greater self-awareness. Some also feel more relaxed given their reduced fertility levels (although pregnancy is still possible during perimenopause).
- *Skin and hair changes:* Due to hormonal changes, it is normal for a woman to experience changes in her skin and hair. Common changes include thinning hair, dry skin, sensitive skin, and increased healing time for cuts and bruises.
- *Sleep issues:* Sleep may be disrupted by hot flashes or night sweats. Sleep may also be erratic without the presence of hot flashes or night sweats. Many women experience wakefulness between 3:00 a.m. and 4:00 a.m.—the period historically referred to as the "witching hour." So if you wake for no apparent reason during this timeframe, trust that you are not alone. Many women are waking at the same time as you!
- *Vaginal issues:* Vaginal atrophy (which is the thinning and drying of the tissues of the vagina and urethra) can be a troubling issue for some women. Caused by a decrease in estrogen production, vaginal atrophy increases a woman's vulnerability to vaginal and urinary infections. For

those who experience a marked decrease in vaginal lubrication and loss of vaginal elasticity, sexual intercourse can become painful.

- *Weight changes*: Weight gain may become a concern (or more of a concern) due to hormonal changes and a slower metabolism. A tendency toward inactivity may also account for some weight gain.

The onset and nature of menopause, just as with perimenopause, is highly individual. As noted, menopause is marked by the absence of a menstrual period for one continuous year. Most women enter menopause in their late forties to early fifties; the average age of onset in the United States is fifty-one. As well, several factors can hasten the onset of menopause. These factors include a history of smoking, chemotherapy, radiation therapy, and being underweight. Women who are overweight may have a later onset of menopause. If the women in your family of origin have a history of early menopause, you may also experience an early menopausal onset.[20]

On a related note, premature menopause (menopause before age forty) occurs in approximately 1 percent of women. Premature menopause may occur due to a condition known as primary ovarian insufficiency (when the ovaries simply do not produce normal levels of female reproductive hormones); this may result from an autoimmune disease or genetic factors.[18] Premature menopause is also associated with smoking, radiation exposure, chemotherapy drugs, or surgery that impairs blood supply to the ovaries.

Finally, surgical menopause may occur in women who have undergone a hysterectomy (surgical removal of the uterus) or oophorectomy (surgical removal of an ovary or ovaries). Women who have a total hysterectomy (removal of uterus) and bilateral oophorectomy (removal of both ovaries) will experience abrupt menopause. In addition, those who have surgical menopause may experience more severe symptoms than those who ease into menopause naturally.

The vast array of symptoms involved in perimenopause and menopause can make these phases quite difficult for many women to bear. Contrary to the popular belief that menopausal women experience more mental health issues than their counterparts, research indicates otherwise. Several studies have found that menopausal women have no greater degree of stressful feelings, anxiety, depression, or anger than women of the same age who are still menstruating.[20] Yet it's truly important to honor the truth that the physical symptoms and life changes that occur during one's menopausal years can be stressful. From the effects of hormonal fluctuations and disturbed sleep to daily stressors and shifting life roles, the rigors of the perimenopausal and menopausal years can take a toll on a woman's mental and emotional health. So whether your symptoms are mild or extreme, it's important to take good care of yourself with effective treatments and lifestyle adjustments that are beneficial for you.

Wisdom Tip 30: Allow Yourself the Gift of Wise Self-Care.

As you move through perimenopause and into menopause, it's important to take good care of yourself. By following the easy-to-use tips outlined below, your quality of life will improve and your joy factor will grow!

Investigate hormone replacement therapy (HRT): Consult your healthcare provider to ascertain if you are a candidate for HRT. Sometimes called ERT (estrogen replacement therapy) and menopausal hormone therapy, various treatments are available and are often very helpful in minimizing perimenopausal symptoms. As well, HRT may protect against osteoporosis. Some HRT treatments contain only one hormone, whereas others contain both estrogen and progesterone. HRT treatment is most commonly prescribed in pill form, but other options include skin patches, vaginal creams, gels, and vaginal rings.

It's important to note that not all women are good candidates for HRT. HRT is not recommended for those who have liver disease, vaginal bleeding issues, or those affected by breast cancer and certain other forms of cancer. Women who have had blood clots, a stroke, or a heart attack are generally not good candidates for HRT. Indeed, there are many notable concerns involved in HRT that include an increased risk of a heart attack, stroke, blood clots, breast cancer, and gallbladder disease. If you are or may be pregnant, consult with your health care provider on the use of HRT.

In general, your unique genetic makeup, personal history, and lifestyle will determine whether or not HRT is right for you. Your health care provider can be an excellent resource in helping you explore your HRT options as well as evaluating the possible risks and benefits. If you are a good candidate for HRT and elect to go this route, it is generally recommended that you take the lowest HRT dose that provides benefits and that you use HRT only as long as necessary. Your primary care provider should consult with you every three to six months to ascertain if HRT is still appropriate or necessary for you.[21]

Investigate alternatives to HRT. Estrogen alternatives, sometimes called synthetic estrogens, may improve vaginal atrophy without increasing a woman's risk for endometrial cancer. Your primary care provider may also recommend non-hormonal treatments, homeopathic remedies, and herbal treatments to relieve various perimenopausal and menopausal symptoms.

Stay abreast of new research: Given the rapid changes in the pharmaceutical and medical worlds, it's important to discuss new treatments with your primary care provider. For example, new research shows that the medication oxybutynin, typically used to treat overactive bladder issues such as incontinence and urinary frequency, can reduce the frequency and intensity of hot flashes for those who are not candidates for HRT. As hot flashes can be more severe for breast cancer survivors than for the general population, and given that breast cancer survivors are among the groups for which HRT is generally not recommended, access to alternative treatments is vital.[22]

Eat healthfully: Treat yourself to a plant-based diet rich in fruits, vegetables, whole grains, legumes, seeds, and nuts. When you use milk products, select those that are non-fat or low-fat. It's important to have a diet rich in omega-3 fatty acids; high levels of omega-3 fatty acids can be found in walnuts, chia seeds, and fish (such as salmon and tuna). Avoid animal products, sugary products, and packaged foods whenever possible. To reduce your risk of osteoporosis, ensure that you add foods to your diet that are high in calcium and vitamin D—both of which may help prevent bone loss.

Some studies show that phytoestrogen extracts (which can be found in soy products such as tofu and soy beans) may reduce symptoms of hot flashes; compelling evidence reflects that they do have positive health effects on lipid panels (e.g., cholesterol) and may reduce heart disease.[23]

> *Note: Vitamin D is a hormone, not a true vitamin. A major dietary source of vitamin D is milk (added per government requirements). Cheese and other milk products are often not fortified with vitamin D. Many plant-based milks (e.g., almond milk and soy milk) are fortified with vitamin D, but the levels do vary. Other foods, such as egg yolks and salmon, are also good sources of vitamin D. Consult your primary care provider to determine if vitamin D supplements are necessary for you.*

Drink hydrating, detoxifying fluids: If you're not drinking a half gallon of water (eight 8-ounce glasses) per day, now is a good time to start. Not only does water keep your skin and body hydrated, but it acts as a cleansing agent for your body. Given that mature skin can feel dry, water is especially important during perimenopause and menopause.

As an added bonus, drinking plenty of water can reduce bloating. When you drink water before and during meals, you're more likely to feel full. When you feel satiated by increasing your water intake during meals, you'll eat less and begin to shed unwanted pounds. Some women find that they are more likely to drink water if it's carbonated, naturally flavored with lemon or fruit, or in the form of hydrating herbal tea. Experiment to discover what is most inviting to you!

Avoid alcohol and caffeine overuse: Research shows that women should consume no more than one alcoholic beverage (5 fluid ounces of wine, 12 fluid ounces of beer, or 1.5 fluid ounces of distilled 80-proof spirits) each day. New research, in fact, questions the often-touted health benefits of even one alcoholic beverage per day.[24] As both alcohol and caffeine can affect mood—frequently increasing irritability—take note if certain symptoms tend to improve when you decrease your intake of alcohol and caffeinated beverages. Alcohol also adds empty calories to your diet, so reducing alcohol intake can have a positive impact on your waistline! If urinary incontinence is an issue, you may find substantial relief by avoiding alcohol and caffeine.

Watch your weight: As obesity is associated with many health conditions (including an increased risk for hot flashes), it's important to maintain a healthy weight. A significant study involved 17,473 women from ages 50 to 79 (who were not using menopausal hormone therapy) where dietary interventions were utilized to increase the women's intake of fruits, vegetables, and whole grains while reducing fat intake. The study found that those who lost at least 10 pounds or 10 percent of their body weight were significantly more likely to eliminate symptoms such as hot flashes and night sweats than those who did not lose weight.[25]

If you are carrying a few extra pounds, losing just 5 percent of your body weight can have powerful health benefits. A recent study found that a loss of 5 percent of one's body weight can improve metabolic function in muscle, fat, and liver tissue while also reducing you risk for heart disease and diabetes.[26] Perimenopausal and menopausal years are the perfect time to reach and maintain a healthy weight. Make positive, steady changes that feel doable to you; small shifts will support you in creating lifelong habits that allow you to care for and enjoy your body!

Exercise often and regularly: Exercise—even in small, fifteen-minute increments—provides many health benefits, including weight loss, stress reduction, improved sleep, and healthier bones, joints, and muscles. Weightbearing exercise such as walking and yoga can be particularly helpful.

When it comes to menopausal symptoms, a year-long study found that only three hours of exercise per week (that's just about twenty-five minutes per day) increased a woman's overall quality of life. The menopausal symptoms of the women in the study also showed significant improvement. Not surprisingly, the control group (the women who did not exercise) found that their menopausal symptoms worsened significantly.[27] You deserve good doses of exercise every week!

Don't smoke: Smoking is associated with many serious health conditions including heart disease, cancer, and increased risk for hot flashes. If you smoke, now is a great time to get the support you need to kick *any* smoking habits!

Protect your sleep: Chronic insomnia can result when sleep is consistently disrupted by hot flashes or night sweats. Your ability to function (physically and mentally) is negatively affected when you don't get sufficient rest. If you lose even one to two hours of sleep for several nights, your ability to function is as compromised as if you'd had no sleep at all for a day or two.[28] Create healthy bedtime routines that support at least seven to eight hours of rest.

A few sleep hygiene tips are key: go to bed at a regular time; keep your bedroom free of electronic devices—particularly those with blue light; have your last meal and beverage several hours before bedtime; reduce distractions like computer use and television as you prepare for bed; investigate the use of calming essential oils, such as lavender and chamomile, to promote sleep; write out "to-do lists" or nagging concerns well before bedtime to help your mind de-clutter and prepare for sleep.

Practice mindfulness: Strive to stay in the moment and notice your thoughts, feelings, and attitudes. Staying in the present will also help you tune in to any foods, substances, activities, or situations that exacerbate perimenopausal and menopausal symptoms. When you slow down to mindfully take note of what doesn't work for you, you'll be more likely to naturally avoid these triggers.

In the same way, mindfulness can help you notice what does work for you—the foods, substances, activities, and situations that make you feel refreshed, healthier, and at your best. By taking note of these positive elements, you can then make choices that will allow you to create more of what works in your life. You might find that you enjoy creating a journal that outlines what makes you feel good—a "love it" list—in order to increase your awareness and promote healthier patterns. For example, if you find that coffee makes you irritable, you might decide to replace coffee with fruity herbal tea. You might find that a certain comfort food makes you feel sluggish and replace it with a different food that leaves you feeling energetic and healthy. (Tart apples are my go-to comfort snack.) If you discover that a brisk, fifteen-minute walk makes you feel energized and cheerful, you can add this activity to your "love it" list.

As well, if you notice that interactions with certain people in your life make you feel positive and loved, you may surely want to add those connections to your "love it" list. This simple, easy-to-follow method allows you to create more joy in your life. All you need do is notice what makes you feel better and do *more* of it. At the same time, notice what doesn't make you feel good and make a deal with yourself to do less of whatever that is. Mindfulness can help you create customized, positive habits that are a win-win for your body, mind, and spirit.

Engage in excellent self-care: You deserve to feel loved and nourished. Good self-care doesn't need to be costly or time-consuming. All you need to do is carve out spots in your day and your week that are dedicated to caring for yourself. These little self-care appointments can be as small as a quiet ten-minute meditation, a relaxing fifteen-minute walk, or a twenty-minute session of body stretching in your living room.

Customize your self-care activities to suit your personal interests and needs. Perhaps you enjoy manicures, knitting, gardening, reading, journal, or creating through art, cooking, or music. If something brings you joy, allow it to become a part of your regular self-care routine. Excellent self-care practices will leave you feeling refreshed, relaxed, and more positive.

When self-care is a top priority, you'll feel better about taking care of whatever is on your to-do list, whether it's tending to the needs of others or managing your own life issues. Self-care isn't selfish—it's absolutely essential to your well-being. Good self-care is a manifestation of strong self-esteem. Through perimenopause, menopause, and beyond, your body, mind, and spirit will thank you for making your needs a priority. You deserve loving selfcare.

Create time with loved ones: From spending time with girlfriends and family to bonding and cuddling with a romantic partner, life simply feels better when we connect with those we love. Whether chatting with compassionate friends about life changes or getting a joyful, reassuring dose of love from one's partner, the mood-elevating benefits of connective time are powerful indeed. So when possible, step away from the computer and remote control and create some face-to-face time with those you love.

Investigating and Normalizing Urinary Incontinence Issues

Let's be honest. It's more than a bit irritating to pee—even a tiny bit—when you cough, sneeze, laugh, exercise, or lift a slightly heavy item. And, truth be told, it's absolutely embarrassing to find that you've "leaked" a little (or a lot) because you couldn't make it to the bathroom in time. In general, it can feel downright uncomfortable not to be in control of your own bodily functions; when personal bodily fluids like urine are involved, the level of discomfort can rise dramatically. If urinary incontinence issues plague you, this section might give you some much deserved comfort and information. Before exploring this topic more fully, I want you to know two important facts: urinary incontinence is extremely common *and* it is very treatable.

The tremendously important topic of bladder control issues deserves to be discussed with honesty and frankness. Stress incontinence and urge incontinence are the two most common types of urinary incontinence in women. Stress incontinence generally results from weak pelvic floor muscles. When pelvic floor muscles are weak, extra stress is placed on the bladder and urethra, and this may result in urine leakage. For those affected by stress incontinence, everyday actions such as laughing, sneezing, coughing, lifting, or exercising can trigger urine leakage in small or large amounts. A recent study found that nearly one-third of those who suffer from urinary incontinence experience a leakage episode almost daily. Seventy-nine percent of the incidents result from sneezing or coughing, 64 percent while attempting to get to a bathroom, 49 percent when laughing, and 37 percent during exercise.[29]

Urge incontinence—also called overactive bladder (OAB)—occurs when bladder muscles squeeze chronically or at the wrong time, and this can cause both leakage and a sense of urgency. Those who suffer from OAB may feel a sudden, intense urge to urinate and may not be able to make it to the bathroom in time. Some women may be able to get to the toilet in time yet may feel the need to urinate more than eight times per day. It's important to note that many women suffer from "mixed" incontinence, in which symptoms of both OAB *and* stress incontinence are experienced.

Clearly, the effects of urinary incontinence conditions can be inconvenient, scary, and highly embarrassing. It's easy to understand why many women with incontinence concerns find themselves building their schedules around their bladder issues. Some women find themselves avoiding outings and social situations solely out of fear of leakage or a concern that a bathroom may not be readily available. As well, many women worry about incontinence-related odor and may feel chronically worried about this issue. Those who suffer from more severe urinary incontinence often dress in layers or wear dark colors to help conceal accidents. Sexual intimacy can also be affected, as some women suffer from bladder leakage during sexual intercourse. Those who experience chronic urinary incontinence issues frequently report having a lower sense of self-esteem, increased anxiety, higher stress levels, and feelings of depression directly related to their bladder condition.

In truth, feelings of embarrassment and shame leave many a woman thinking that she is the only one suffering from urinary incontinence issues. In fact, according to a recent study, women are so hesitant to talk about their urinary incontinence issues that only 28 percent of women age 50–64 discuss the issue with their health care provider. This is terribly unfortunate given that 43 percent of women in the study's 50–64 group and 51 percent of those in the 65–80 age group reported urinary incontinence in the past year.[29] Another study (one that involved 3,000 women from 42 to 64 years of age and the analysis of nine years of data) determined that *68 percent* of women experience urinary incontinence issues at least one time per month.[30] To bring this last statistic home, imagine this: If you're in a room of ten women whose ages range from 42 to 64, nearly seven of these women have experienced some form of bladder leakage at least once in the past month. If you've felt alone in having urinary incontinence issues, you now know that you've plenty of good company.

Given the profound statistics just mentioned, it's time that we take women's bladder control issues out of the closet and into the light of awareness and normalcy where they belong. And to be fair and straightforward, urinary incontinence doesn't affect only mature women; it affects males and females across a wide range of age groups. For example, overactive bladder is one of the most common bladder issues; OAB affects about 33 million Americans. Approximately 40 percent of females and 30 perfect of males have overactive bladder symptoms.[31] In fact, one large study found that OAB without urge incontinence was *more* common in men than women across all age groups.[32] Given that many people don't reach out for medical care, the real numbers of those who live with conditions such as OAB are thought to be much higher. So whether you're in the company of men or women, trust that you are not the only one who may have a sudden, uncontrollable urge to urinate, a bit of leakage, or the need to run to the restroom more frequently than you'd like. In fact, you might already feel quite a bit better just knowing that urinary incontinence is a common human condition—not just your private, secret problem.

It's important to note that urinary incontinence is not considered a "normal" part of aging but rather a heath condition that can be treated. Urinary incontinence commonly results from pregnancy, childbirth, and menopause and in generally attributed to weakened pelvic floor muscles that support the bladder, urethra, uterus, and bowels. If the muscles that support the urinary tract become weak or damaged, the extra pressure on the bladder and urethra may cause leakage. As well, a female's urethra is shorter than a male's, so there is less muscle to keep the urine in place. Other causes of urinary incontinence include: being overweight, bladder and urinary tract infections, caffeine use, certain medications (e.g., diuretics), constipation, currently smoking, surgery involving reproductive organs, and nerve damage resulting from diabetes, multiple sclerosis, and childbirth.[33, 34]

Many primary care providers do not openly ask their clients if they are experiencing incontinence issues. This is highly unfortunate and is an area where change is certainly needed. As women are often embarrassed or ashamed to discuss this personal topic, primary care providers can be excellent role models in opening up communication on these common and treatable concerns. Yet if your primary care provider is not leading the way, strive to be your own advocate—and a role model—in discussing your concerns in a straightforward way. Remember that you are not alone! Your quality of life and overall health are worth any twinges of initial embarrassment. It's also important to acknowledge that many women feel more comfortable talking with female health care providers about incontinence issues. This makes perfect sense; feel free to request a female health care provider if you feel more comfortable discussing these intimate issues with another woman. Do what feels right for you.

Many treatments are available for bladder incontinence issues. When you talk with your primary care provider, insist on exploring and discovering the ideal treatment for your situation. Both surgical and non-surgical treatment options are available. A few of the most common include medication called imipramine (originally an anti-depressant, but also used for stress incontinence), pelvic floor exercises (described subsequently), biofeedback, and bladder retraining. Botox can be a highly effective treatment for OAB. Laser and radio frequency treatments applied to the interior of the vagina may be appropriate for stress incontinence. Vaginal sling surgery is a more invasive option that utilizes a natural or synthetic material to support the urethra (the bladder neck). As surgical procedures involve risks, it is important to discuss the possible risks and benefits with your health care provider.

Wisdom Tip 31: Address Bladder Issues with Awareness and Compassion.

If you've been suffering from bladder incontinence, trust that you don't need to suffer any longer. The outline below will offer you some helpful strategies and tips.[33, 35]

- *Lose that extra weight:* If you're overweight, strive to shed some of those unwanted pounds. Excess weight puts greater pressure on your bladder and supportive muscles, and the extra pressure can lead to bladder control issues.
- *Do your Kegels:* Also known as pelvic floor muscle exercises, Kegel exercises can often help with stress incontinence by strengthening the muscles in the pelvic floor. First, isolate your pelvic floor muscles; you can do this by trying to stop your urination flow mid-stream. It might also be helpful to imagine yourself sitting on a flat surface and lifting a marble with your pelvic floor muscles. Once

you've identified your pelvic floor muscles, you're ready to begin your Kegel routine.

When your bladder is *empty*, tighten your pelvic floor muscles for five seconds and then relax them for five seconds; repeat this exercise five times per day for the first day or two. When you are comfortable with this routine, increase to three sets of contracting for ten seconds and relaxing for ten seconds. Strive to work up to (and maintain) three sets of ten to fifteen seconds for three to four sessions per day. You can do your Kegels nearly any time—while in your car, at your desk, as you read, or when you're watching television. Take care to avoid flexing the muscles in your buttocks, thighs, and abdomen; focus on your pelvic floor muscles. Also, be sure to breathe freely—rather than unconsciously holding your breath—as you do your Kegels.

Once you get used to doing Kegels, they will become an instinctive, daily part of your routine. Your bladder will thank you for being committed to strengthening your pelvic floor muscles!

Fun fact: Pelvic floor strengthening exercises are also known to increase sexual pleasure; you might consider this just another motivating reason to do your daily Kegel exercises. Yes!

- *Treat constipation:* If you suffer from constipation, strive to eat more fiber, drink more liquids, and utilize other healthy treatments to improve your bowel movement's regularity. Besides making you feel heavy and clogged, constipation can worsen urinary incontinence.

Personal tip: Check with your primary care physician to see if daily magnesium supplements (which often benefit bowel regularity, as well as muscles and bones) are appropriate for you.

- *If you smoke, give it up:* Smoking has been linked to many health conditions, one of which is urinary incontinence.
- *Watch what you drink:* Alcohol and caffeine may worsen urinary incontinence. As some women may be affected by carbonated beverages, take note if carbonated drinks impact any incontinence issues you may have.
- *Notice foods that activate bladder issues:* Slow down to explore the foods that are triggering for you. Common bladder irritants include apples, chocolate, citrus juice, citrus fruits, corn syrup, cranberries, spicy foods, honey, milk, tomatoes, vinegar, sugar, and artificial sweeteners. If certain foods increase your bladder concerns, remember that you have plenty of other healthy options.
- *Don't limit your intake of water:* Many women with incontinence concerns find themselves drinking less water to avoid leakage and frequent trips to the bathroom. Unfortunately, limiting your water intake results in more concentrated urine in the bladder; this can be highly irritating to bladder tissue.

    A lack of hydration is not beneficial for your body as a whole; your body's vital organs and tissues need plenty of water to function at their optimal level. Frequent urination and leakage are less likely to occur if you drink pure water rather than caffeinated beverages or sugary drinks.
- *Use pads and protective undergarments designed for bladder issues.* Many women resort to using menstrual pads, yet these are often not as helpful as those specifically created for urine leakage.
- *Retrain your bladder:* Because the bladder is controlled by muscles, it can be trained. Patience and persistence are key when creating new bladder routines that will help prevent leakage and emergencies. Bladder control training is a process that gradually teaches you to hold in urine for slightly longer and longer periods of time.

A few basics include going to the bathroom as soon as you wake and then adhering to a set urination schedule throughout the day—even if the urge to urinate is not present. Nighttime trips to the toilet are on an as-needed basis. Your primary care provider can help you determine the bladder retraining routine that is ideal for you. While your bladder is being retrained, don't be shy about wearing protective pads. Patience is key!

When our bodies don't function the way we want them to, even the simplest aspects of daily life can be distressing. It is my hope that this section has left you feeling more aware, less alone, and more empowered as a woman. You now have solid information that can truly help you if you've been suffering in silence from bladder issues. As well, what you've learned may allow you to support any loved ones in your life who may be struggling with similar concerns.

Sexuality and the Maturing Woman

Now we're moving to one of my favorite topics—healthy sexuality. Although sexuality is a basic part of humanity, it is (like far too many important topics) habitually not discussed with the respectful honesty it deserves. So prepare yourself for a healthy dose of truthfulness and fun as we delve into the world of sexuality.

Some women fully embrace their sexuality, others find it an off-putting aspect of life, and many find themselves somewhere between these two poles. Like everything in life, it's your personal preference and truth that matter most, yet many women haven't had the opportunity or desire to openly explore their own sexuality. This is tremendously unfortunate, for our sexuality is a vital part of who we are as women.

Given society's mixed messages, some women find themselves fearful of being too sexual or not sexual enough. Conflicting expectations tell us that we should be virginal yet somehow secretly wild and passionate. At one turn we're told to embrace our sexuality, and then we go around the corner to discover that our own sexuality is being shamed. Although we've made incredible progress in the last few decades, mixed messages are all too common. As well, there are still segments of the population who disparage those who are not "sexually mainstream"; many women who are bi-sexual, lesbian, or trans are often secretly met with disdain. When you add in certain religious beliefs, the topic of sexuality becomes even more complicated. It's no wonder that many women (and men) of all ages find themselves confused when it comes to sexuality.

As if sexuality isn't an already taboo topic in our society, you might have noticed that it's particularly off-limits for older adults. It's as though our society sees delightful sexuality as somehow being reserved for those in their youth—almost as if older adults should no longer like sex or even *have* sex. I find this absolutely bizarre, for humans are—by nature—sexual beings. Sexuality is not confined to one phase in life; sexuality is certainly an aspect of life to be enjoyed through one's entire adult life. Of course, areas of sexuality will shift and change; that's the very nature of life. Yet where one aspect of sexuality might fade, another can be allowed to rise. Now that you're stepping into a new phase in your life, this may be the *perfect* time to experiment and embrace whatever feels good to you (even if it is new or unfamiliar) in order to create greater well-being and joy in your life.

If you find comfort in knowing where you stand compared to others—in terms of your age group, sex, or relationship status—statistics can provide wonderful information. In general, research data can make us feel less alone in our struggles; numbers can provide the solace of knowing that others share our concerns and experiences. In a similar vein, statistics often provide comforting reassurance of normalcy; pressing concerns lessen with the realization that one's situation or issue is somewhere in the "ordinary" range. In addition, some utilize such data as motivation for personal change, particularly when they are experiencing distress or undesirable consequences as a result of mental, emotional, or situational issues. As you read the following paragraphs, strive to avoid judgment and allow yourself to utilize whatever information speaks to you in the most constructive ways.

Let's start off with a few facts that illuminate the frisky, sexual aspect of older adulthood. In a recent survey of men and women age 65 and over, 76 percent believed that sexual intimacy is important in romantic relationships, regardless of age; 84 percent of men held this belief, whereas only 69 percent of women felt similarly. Over half of the respondents reported that sex was important to their overall quality of life; men (70 percent) were more likely to hold this belief than women (40 percent). Sexually active adults were far more likely to report that sex was important for their quality of life than those who were not sexually active (83 percent compared to 35 percent). Sixty-five percent of respondents reported being interested in sex, with younger respondents age 65–70 being nearly twice as likely to be interested in sex when compared to those age 76–80. *Almost 75 percent of the older adults surveyed reported being satisfied with their sex lives.* Women were more likely than men to report being "extremely" or "very" satisfied. And those with a romantic partner and those in better health were more likely to report feeling satisfied with their sex lives.[37]

With the above statistics for the over-sixty-five population in our heads, let's look at some data for younger demographics. One recent study found that American adults in their twenties have sex, on average, eighty times per year (about 1.5 times per week), whereas those in their sixties reported an average of twenty times per year (roughly 1.5 times per month).[38] A recent study investigating sexual interest found that for those age 16–74, only 15 percent of men reported lacking sexual interest compared to slightly over 34 percent of women.[39] As to frequency of sex and how it relates to overall relationship satisfaction, another study determined that sex is certainly associated with a sense of well-being in relationships, but that noteworthy benefits don't accrue after a certain level. In short, sex one time per week predicts greater well-being, but sex more than once per week does not significantly increase well-being for those in relationships.[40]

Now, let's explore some interesting statistics focused solely on women. One female-only study found that 61 percent of women age forty and older (with a median age of sixty-seven) reported being satisfied with their sex lives. For these women—90 percent of whom reported being in good or excellent health—more frequent arousal, lubrication, and orgasm were associated with feeling emotionally close during sex. Half of the women reported sexual activity within the past month, and one-third of the women reported low or absent sexual desire. Two-thirds of the sexually active women reported being moderately or very satisfied with their sex lives, and about half of the sexually inactive women reported the same. Interestingly, the study's conclusion noted that sexual satisfaction increased with a woman's age and was not contingent upon being sexually active; clearly, it's a woman's sense of being content—her state of mind—that makes all the difference.[41]

What's *really* going on inside a woman when it comes to sex? Let's delve into a few sexy statistics on women's sexual behaviors, interests, and pleasure. The data—gathered from women age eighteen and over across the United States—may leave you laughing, curious, and feeling not so alone. As you read, feel free to imagine what you want more of (or less of) in your own sexual realm. You might even wish to use what you are learning as fuel to talk with your partner, explore more of what interests you, and gain a greater understanding of your own sexuality. For your reading pleasure, below are the spicy, women-only stats[42]:

- 60 percent of women want *more* sexual intercourse.
- 64 percent of women want more sensual touching.
- 60 percent of women believe their sex lives could be better.
- 46 percent of women believe they are at their sexual prime—regardless of their age.
- 60 percent of women over age eighteen try new experiences in the bedroom. Note that women age forty-five to

fifty-five lead the way with *89 percent* engaging in sexual experimentation. For those who like experimenting, this is great news. For those who want to get more playfully experimental, feel free to get behind adding sex toys, new positions, and healthy products (lubricants, oils, and sensation-enhancers) to your sexual experiences. You go, girl!

- 54 percent of women find sex more pleasurable as they age. (70 percent attribute this to being more comfortable with their body, and 50 percent note that it's a result of spending more time with their partner.)
- 46 percent of women felt that sex worsened as they aged. (70 percent cited decreased sex drive and 46 percent noted vaginal dryness and pain as the cause.)
- The four most common reasons for avoiding sex included weight concerns (48 percent), digestive issues (16 percent), bladder problems (11 percent), and the good, old-fashioned headache (10 percent).

When it comes right down to it, what women *really* want is to find healthy pleasure and contentment within their world of sexuality. Whether in a romantic relationship or not, whatever your sexual preference may be, a healthy relationship with your own sexuality is vital. Knowing what you want—and reaching for it—is half the fun.

It's important to note that romantic relationships tend to thrive in the sexual realm when partners are matched up on sexual desire. It's common for sexual encounters to be fun and frequent during the early stages of a relationship, yet one or both partners can drop the ball when it comes to keeping sexuality alive. Simply put, this can put a heavy strain on the relationship—particularly when one partner is craving sexual intimacy and the other is indifferent or uninterested. Barring significant health issues or severe life stressors (e.g., death of a loved one, new job, or severe financial hardship), there's no reason for partners to let sexual intimacy fade or diminish. In fact, of the three primary relationship stressors, two are directly related to sex—work-related stress is the top relationship stressor, and being too tired for sex and having low sex drive come in second and third.[43] It's unfortunate that many women find themselves in situations where sex (which is meant to be naturally pleasurable and connective in nature) is an ongoing relationship stressor.

Of course, there are times when a natural dip in sexual intimacy occurs, such as when a partner feels tired, sick, or over-stressed. Yet when sexual intimacy is alive and well in a relationship, these dips are more of the exception rather than the rule. Rather than putting energy into healthy sexuality, some partners end up getting consumed with television, computer time, or cell phone use; this affects the couple's level of connection and intimacy. Indeed, a couple's sex life is as important as exercising, engaging in personal hobbies, and even eating dinner. Sexual intimacy is, in truth, a key source of physical and emotional connection within a romantic relationship. In fact, in monogamous relationships, sexual intercourse is the one thing that a woman can't get anywhere *but* from her partner. So if one partner is withholding sex from the other, that partner is creating extra stress—and disharmony—in the relationship.

If you find that you and your partner don't have matching libido levels, it's important to talk about the issue. First, consult your health care providers to rule out medical issues. Those who find a medical basis for low libido (e.g., low hormone levels) often benefit from medication. Note that medications like Viagra *don't* increase libido and sexual interest; they simply increase the ability to get and maintain an erection once aroused. That said, for both men and women who have naturally low libido or have psychological issues (e.g., controlling or passive-aggressive behaviors), it's important to talk openly about creating new and healthy patterns. If one person has a high libido and their partner is not particularly interested in sex, a middle ground can be created. For example, if one partner wants sex daily and the other would prefer sex once a month, the couple can negotiate sexual intimacy time once per week.

There are also times when psychotherapy or sex therapy is truly necessary to help a couple connect and get to the bottom of troublesome issues. Healthy communication opens the door to connective intimacy, whereas closing down and avoiding issues creates chronic resentment. Remember, it's natural for some women to have a racing libido and passionate craving for sex, while others (from teenage years forward) may have never found sex very compelling. These natural variations occur in all genders and across all age ranges. The goal is to work with your partner to have a consistent and healthy sexual relationship that allows both parties to feel seen, loved, and pleasured.

Communication about all topics—including sexuality—is absolutely essential between romantic partners. Many couples are affected by issues that could be addressed and healed if given attention with loving compassion. For example, some women feel unloved and unwanted by their partners as a result of diminished sexual intimacy. Sometimes, indeed, a lack of attraction is at work, yet there are many times that a partner is simply stressed or distracted. If the issue were talked about openly, partners could find connection, both from talking about the issue and then creating romantic time that would feel healing and stress-relieving to both!

As another example, erectile dysfunction can be a sore spot for many couples. Erectile dysfunction (a male's inability to maintain an erection sufficient enough to allow sexual pleasure for both partners) is a common condition that begins to affect many men during their forties; sexual function often decreases markedly after age fifty. Although erectile dysfunction is a medical condition, the situation (if not openly addressed) may be misperceived by the other partner as a lack of desire or interest. Often, both partners are distressed and suffering—the male may secretly feel ashamed and humiliated, while the woman may feel hurt and rejected.

As one dear friend told me, "My former partner attached his impotence to the size of my rear. Literally. Then I lost a bunch of weight, and his problem did not get better. I gained all that weight back. It was attached to another person's ego instead of my heart. I'm in a place where I've lost all that weight again because of my commitment to my well-being."

Sadly, such stories are far more common than not. The unnecessary shame surrounding impotence (and other sexual issues) is too frequently projected outward onto one's partner. By openly talking about erectile dysfunction, increased understanding can lead to greater awareness and the use of helpful techniques that aid with sexual functioning. Healthy communication is a win-win; when we talk kindly and openly with our partner about our concerns, feelings such as embarrassment and rejection are decreased, while connective feelings of understanding and compassion are increased. What could be better than that?

Wisdom Tip 32: Embrace the Delights of Healthy Sexuality.

Let's explore a few tips for increasing healthy sexuality in your life.[44]

- Get to know what pleasures you: Explore your body to notice what feels right—your most sensitive areas, the level of pressure you like, and the positions that feel right to you. What may have felt great when you were twenty or thirty may no longer do the trick for you. For those who like experimenting, different avenues can be explored with well-trained sexuality professionals, such as tantric sex experts.
- Communicate openly with your partner: A healthy relationship allows for open discussion on all issues—including what one does and does not prefer in the bedroom. If your partner is shy or sensitive about "getting it wrong in the bedroom," gentle suggestions, the guiding of hands, or the thoughtful introduction of sex toys may be helpful.
- Set up and maintain date nights with your partner: Whether once or twice a week, create romantic time where you can relax and play with your partner.

This time can be used for massages, baths, kissing, cuddling—or more.

- Take the pressure off by removing orgasm or intercourse as the primary goal: Gentle caressing of the entire body— and the erogenous zones—offers significant pleasure in its own right. Once the pressure is off and partners feel more connected, nature usually takes its own course.
- Create romance with bubble baths and warm showers: Bathing with your loved one can be both relaxing and bonding. Take care with bath products, as some can irritate the increasingly thin and sensitive vaginal tissues.
- Have sex more often! On a physiological level, frequent intercourse is healthy for both females and males. Frequent sex increases blood flow to sexual organs and keeps tissues healthier. (For men, frequent ejaculation protects the prostate.) Of course, regular sex improves connection, mood, and outlook!
- Allow sufficient arousal time: Slow down your sexual interludes to allow the body plenty of time to create its own lubricants. Although the addition of other lubricants can sometimes be necessary, a woman's body typically begins to flow with natural lubrication if given sufficient time and gentle stimulation.
- Invest in top-quality lubricants: Although lubricants can be wonderful additions to one's sex life at any age, they can be particularly helpful if your vaginal tissue is dry and thin. As vaginal lubrication often decreases during perimenopause and menopause, it's important to invest in high-quality products that are not drying or irritating to sensitive vaginal tissues. Organic products are a great option.
- Avoid drugs and alcohol: Many drugs and alcohol actually slow down the body's response time. As well, libido-fighting drowsiness often results; this can lead to decreased sexual interest and impaired sexual abilities.

- Exercise frequently: Physical activity improves mood, energy level, and body image—all of which may increase one's interest in sex.
- Do your pelvic floor exercises: Remember those Kegel exercises? Not only will they increase your bladder control by strengthening your pelvic floor muscles, but they may do wonders for you in the realm of sexual pleasure.
- Give up smoking: Your ability to become sexually aroused can be affected by smoking. Cigarette smoking can reduce vaginal blood flow and decrease the effects of estrogen.
- Get playful: If what you're doing in the bedroom isn't working, explore new territory. Whether you visit a sweet sex shop or take a look at toys online, feel free to experiment with your sexuality. From vibrators and dildos to sexy lingerie and sex board games, you'll find many options to energize your sex life.
- Keep your sexy new routines going: It can be easy to slip back into old habits, so make a commitment with your partner (or yourself if you are single) to keep your sex life fresh and alive. Just as you wouldn't ignore getting groceries or filling up your car with gas, your sex life deserves to be a top priority.
- Visit your health care provider: If troubling issues arise that affect your sexuality, reach out to your health care provider right away. Whether you are suffering from painful vaginal dryness, night sweats, lack of sleep, or other issues, ask your health care provider for personalized tips, guidance, support, and medication when necessary.

This phase of your life can be so full and rich. Indeed, it can be a time of wildness, exploration, and new beginnings. With your physical, psychological, and spiritual health in mind, allow yourself to explore your sexuality and do more of whatever gives you joy.

Let me touch on one more important aspect of your sexual health—the often-scary and disconcerting realm of sexually transmitted diseases (STDs). Whether you are married, single, monogamous, polygamous, heterosexual, bi-sexual, lesbian, sexually active, or sexually inactive, it's important to be aware of STDs. No segment of the population is immune from STDs. As such, it's always a good idea to have an STD screening done during one's annual exam. If you or your partner have had more than one sexual partner, it's absolutely vital that you have routine STD screenings on the schedule recommended by your health care provider. Strive to be at peace with this aspect of your sexuality, for when it comes to STDs, most women have had to face an STD issue in their lifetime.

The level of shame that comes with having an STD can be enormous. Many women feel defective and unlovable as a result of finding that they have an STD. Yet, unfortunately, STDs are a fact of life. If you are a woman with an STD, trust that you are certainly not alone. Having an STD is not something to feel guilty or embarrassed about. You are, however, responsible for good self-care and honest communication with your partner(s), as well as obligated to take responsible, protective measures when engaging in sexual activity. If you have an STD, let new partners know of your condition before having sex. If your existing partner doesn't know that you have an STD, discuss the situation openly and honestly.

The term STD encompasses a variety of sexually transmitted infections caused by bacteria, viruses, or parasites. *It's very important to note that STDs can be transmitted by oral, anal, and vaginal sexual contact, not just by traditional sexual intercourse alone.* Some STDs can be transmitted in non-sexual contact via bodily fluids (e.g., shared toothbrushes, razors, or other personal hygiene products.) To take some of the fear out of this STD issue, below is an outline of several common STDs. If you are concerned about STDs, reach out to your primary care provider for a complete list of STDs and STD issues.[45, 46]

- Human papillomavirus (HPV), the most common STD, is an infection that can cause warts in various parts of the body. Although HPV usually clears up on its own, untreated HPV can lead to cervical cancer and other forms of cancer in both women and men. HPV affects one in four people in the United States. Although a vaccine is available, it is administered to young women through age twenty-six.
- Chlamydia, which may not cause symptoms, is a common STD caused by a bacteria. Chlamydia is easy to treat with appropriate antibiotics.
- Gonorrhea is a bacterial infection that may lead to infertility if it is not treated. This STD, once diagnosed, responds well to proper antibiotic treatment.
- Syphilis, another STD caused by bacteria, usually begins as a painful sore and can be spread by sexual activity. Left untreated, syphilis can cause permanent damage. Syphilis can be treated with appropriate antibiotics.
- Hepatitis B is caused by a virus and can be spread through sexual activity and by sharing personal hygiene items, such as toothbrushes and razors. This virus can cause liver disease. Although there is no cure for Hepatitis B, management treatments are available. A vaccine to prevent Hepatitis B is also available.
- Genital herpes is another common STD caused by a virus; it is marked by outbreaks of painful, blistery lesions. Although there is no cure, anti-viral treatments are available.
- HIV, the virus that causes AIDs, is yet another worrisome STD. Although there is no cure for HIV or AIDs, treatments to help manage the condition are available.

Some STDs have obvious symptoms like foul-smelling vaginal discharge, itching, or burning. Other STDs can be non-symptomatic and even lie dormant in a woman's body for years. If you haven't been checked for STDs, or if you've been checked in the past and have had any new sexual partners or a sexual partner who is not monogamous, ask your primary care provider to order the necessary tests.

Wisdom Tip 33: Enter the Realm of Dating with Wise Awareness.

As many women in their fifties and beyond are heading out into the dating world after divorce or the death of a partner, it's important to be savvy during this often-scary adventure. When it comes to your body and your sexuality, I want you to feel as informed and empowered as you do in all others areas of your life. So if your journey takes you into dating, marriage, and sexual activity, know that you can navigate this new territory with grace and joy.

- Make an appointment with your primary care provider to discuss your sexual health; request that you be screened for STDs.
- If you have an STD, let prospective partners know about the condition prior to engaging in any sexual activity. Discuss the issue openly, honestly, and unapologetically. If your prospective partner is put off by the issue, don't take it personally. Take any rebuff as a sign that you are meant to move onward.
- If you do have an STD and an accepting partner, make sure to consistently use protection (e.g., condoms). Protective practices can become a part of foreplay!
- Don't let yourself be defined by an STD. Know that you are far more than any condition you might have.
- Require a recent STD screening from every potential sexual partner. The health of your body is on the line, so stand up for yourself when it comes to knowing the STD history of an individual that you are considering as a sexual partner. If the individual balks at having testing done or offering you current proof, consider this a major

red flag—a sign of clear disrespect—and smile joyfully as you walk away. You and your health deserve to be treated with absolute honor and respect.

Doesn't it feel good to know so much about your body? Doesn't it feel absolutely terrific to be informed and in love with all of who you are? As you venture forward into these next years of your life, embrace your sexuality—your entire sexual being—with joy. You, lovely lady, are a gift to the world. As you shine with delight at being comfortable in your own gorgeous skin, your self-love and self-acceptance will be a radiant guide for others.

Memory Changes

Oh, did I forget to cover something? There's one more important topic, but I can't remember what it is. Hmmmm . . . Well, that's an aging brain for you! On a serious note, it's important that we delve—just a bit—into memory issues. Indeed, many women in their fifties and beyond struggle with not feeling "with it."

Just a few days ago, I was chatting with a lively group of women whose ages ranged from twenty-five to eighty-five. One vibrant woman in her sixties noted how difficult it was to get any project done given the many trips she made back and forth to get one object. I smiled as she noted, "I go upstairs to get something, but by the time I get there I've forgotten what I needed. Then I go back downstairs, finally remember what I wanted to get, and then have to do the process all over again. Seriously, it's become a form of exercise!" The other women smiled and commiserated—even the youngest one. Another woman added, "I'm glad it's not just me. I do that same thing several times a day—more often than I'd like to admit. Sometimes I think I'm losing my mind."

If this sounds familiar to you, you might have found yourself wondering if you are simply forgetful or if you've entered the realm of dementia. On a positive note, many perceived memory issues are actually the result of busyness and distraction. A mentor once offered me a somewhat simplistic way to help clients differentiate between serious memory issues and a distracted mind: If you go to the store and forget where you parked your car, it's likely that you were simply distracted when you were parking and didn't notice significant markers. If, however, you go to the store and can't remember how you got there or where you are, now *that's* a memory issue.

Yet it is true that memory does change with time. Our minds can become increasingly filled with to-do lists, worries, and life concerns. When this occurs, we tend to be less mindful of what we are doing in the current moment, whether it is where we put our car keys or what we've done with our cell phone. Slowing down and staying mindful may offer the perfect "cure" for your memory issues. Regardless of one's age, memory can be temporarily affected by many issues, including the following: amount of sleep, diet, stress level, emotional state (e.g., anger and fear), anxiety, and mental health issues (e.g., chronic depression). Memory can also be affected by worrying about memory—the more you stress about memory issues, the more you might be spending your energy on worry rather than paying attention to the present moment.

Wisdom Tip 34: Enhance Your Memory Mindfully.

It's normal to have minor fluctuations in memory each day. To keep your memory in top form, try these tips:

- Eat a healthy diet with plenty of fresh fruits and veggies; organic blueberries are a powerful brain food.
- Keep your brain and body active with a variety of physical and mental exercises and activities.
- Get plenty of sleep, generally recommended to be seven to eight hours per night.
- Make lists. There's no shame—and certainly a lot of power—in creating to-do lists for daily activities, shopping, and commitments. Lists leave your brain free to

tend to other tasks, and you'll save yourself plenty of stress, worry, and trips to the store.

- Keep important items in one place. If you've a special spot for your keys, phone, and other significant items, you are far less likely to lose them.
- Stay mindful rather than stressing over your memory or telling yourself that you're going crazy. Simply slow down to stay in the present moment, focus on what's important, and enjoy what you're doing.
- Multi-tasking leads to diminished focus and inattention. Strive to stay focused on one task at a time.
- Connect with others socially. Your brain will stay younger when you engage in activities that keep you connected and feeling joyful.
- Play! Your memory and attitude will benefit when you embrace opportunities to engage in playful activities with people of all ages. Whether you have grandchildren or other little ones in your life, you and the youngsters will surely benefit from increased play time.

Many women in their fifties and sixties begin to worry about "getting" dementia. Dementia (which isn't a specific disease but rather a cluster of symptoms) is diagnosed when the symptoms affect memory, cognitive abilities, and social functioning to a degree that daily functioning is impaired. Dementia most frequently occurs in a progressive fashion and has many underlying causes, such as vascular disorders or Alzheimer's disease. Although symptoms of dementia vary widely, common cognitive changes include: confusion and disorientation, difficulty with planning and organizing, difficulty handling complex tasks, difficulty communicating or finding words, and difficulty reasoning or problem-solving. As well, friends and family often notice memory loss issues and register concern. Psychological changes are also associated with dementia and may include: agitation, paranoia, anxiety, personality changes, depression, inappropriate behavior, and hallucinations. If memory issues plague you, it's important to reach out to your primary care provider and a specialist for a thorough evaluation.

You might now feel somewhat reassured by knowing that memory issues are common and can often be attributed to lifestyle factors. So the next time you lose those car keys or forget where you put your glasses, take heart. It's likely that you're simply too busy and distracted. Trust that you can take steps now to support good brain health and keep your memory in top form for many years to come.

It's been a joy and a pleasure exploring such a wide range of important and sensitive topics with you. It is my heartfelt hope that you now understand and appreciate your amazing body just a little bit more. It's my prayer that you take steps to make whatever changes are necessary to improve your health and overall well-being. I know you have this power within you. I know that—one step at a time—you can move toward the healthy lifestyle that you deserve. And, in the end, it is your joy that is most important. From the food that nourishes your body and mind to exercise habits that strengthen and protect your entire being, I want to support you in radiating from the inside out. When you look in the mirror, I pray you see a joyful, luminous woman looking back at you. This is you. This is me. This is us. This is healthy, joy-filled womanhood.

CHAPTER 4

Tuning In to Your Relationships and Roles

*F*rom your twenties through your mid-life years, you may have found yourself buffeted about by constant change. Indeed, during these full decades of life, change may have been the only constant in your life. Women can be pros at adapting to change—often at great hidden expense to themselves. Although some women can make the shifts from one role and life stage to another seem ever so easy, these busy years of life often take a heavy, unconscious toll on the body and psyche.

To make everything run as smoothly as possible, you may have raced full speed ahead through each day without awareness of yourself, your relationships, and your many roles in life. Like many women, you may have simply done what needed to be done to get through each day. With a focus on pleasing others—making everyone as happy as could be—you may have lost touch with yourself.

It's quite possible that you simply didn't have time to ponder the meaning and nature of your own life.

That makes perfect sense, for early adulthood schedules are filled with an ever-changing variety of tasks. In the course of her days, a woman often finds herself immersed in an exhausting array of roles and responsibilities. Your standard go-to list might have included juggling some mixture of the following: friends, dating, work duties, bills, cooking, the needs of a significant other, family issues, pregnancy, new babies, growing children, financial issues, carpools, dance lessons, daycare, school field trips, career changes, health issues, soccer games, laundry, work schedules, car repairs, shopping, volunteering, in-law concerns, doctor visits, birthday parties, homework, school schedules, busy vacations, relationship hiccups, home repairs, holiday events, and more. Clearly, schedules like this don't leave a great deal of time for quiet introspection and soul-searching. Yet now, for the first time in decades, you may be pausing to ask yourself questions like: "Who am I?"; "What state are my relationships in?"; and "What have I done with my life?"

The later decades of life provide a most beautiful opportunity to consciously explore the questions and feelings that might be welling up inside of you. By avoiding the tendency to push such thoughts or emotions back down, you set the stage for exploring the wealth of internal information that is begging for your attention. As you look on your prior roles and relationships with compassionate awareness, you can use the wisdom you garner to find incredible selfappreciation and liberation.

The Roles of Youth: And So It Flew By in a Blur

If you're like many women, you spent the first two decades of your life exploring, wondering, fretting, and doing your best to find your place in the world. You may have struggled with your place in your family of origin. If you were one of the lucky ones, you may have fit in and felt supported, accepted, and right at home. If not, you may have felt like a foreign object—the proverbial ugly duckling, baby bird without a nest, or postman's daughter. Indeed, I can now laugh at my mother's constant insistence that I was found on the doorstep in a basket. As the ninth, precocious child in a teeming brood of ten, I often wondered if her words were true. Indeed, it would have explained why I often felt as if I were an oddity or unwanted—as if I somehow didn't *really* belong.

You may have had similar wonderings deep inside yourself. You may have found yourself questioning why you weren't daddy's princess, mommy's favorite, your siblings' friend, or your grandparents' darling. You may have secretly wondered if you were really loved or really wanted at all. As you grew, you might have accepted your roles or curiously explored what it meant to be a little girl, a daughter, and a sister. Depending on how those around you responded to your presence and your questioning mind, you may have felt ease or discomfort in your various roles as a growing child. If your natural inquisitiveness was dismissed or quashed, those early seeds of confused curiosity may have stayed with you through your early years of life and beyond. Indeed, unanswered wonderings often silently follow us through life as we search for where and how we fit in. Although the many curiosities and demands of youth might busy us with their distractions, these secret thoughts do not magically disappear. They get pushed down as we begin the journey away from family and into the world of friends and school.

And so, you may have spent the first and second decades of life traipsing around in a world that was sometimes delightful and often tremendously confusing. As you explored the world outside of home, you likely formed early friendships and experienced first crushes that pressed at your heart. All the while, your brain soaked in vast amounts of information about the world and your place within it. Your sense of self continued to form as you experienced both rejections and successes at school, among friends, and at home.

In one way or another, you unconsciously were drawn to play various roles. Perhaps you experimented with being a girly-girl, a tomboy, or a blend of gender roles that felt interesting, unfamiliar, or very comfortable. You may have been subjected to labels, such as the "smart one," "pretty one," "loner," "drama queen," "good girl," "bad girl," "sensitive child," "dummy," "geek," or "ugly duckling." You may have bought into the labels or you might have thrown off their weight in disdain. You may have unconsciously adopted certain roles and ways of being due to the labels cast on you, or you might have consciously forged ahead to determine your own path. Some of this may have come easily and naturally to you, or it might have taken nearly everything you had to hold up your head and do what you needed to do to get by. There is no right or wrong in any of this; it is the truth and the nature of what happens during the first formative decades of life.

Then, all of a sudden, you likely found yourself plopped into the independence of young adulthood. As you became acclimated to subsisting outside of your parents' home, you may have found yourself both delighted and bewildered once again—this time by the interplay of your newfound autonomy and the demands of adult life. Your late teens and twenties may have found you playing the field, exploring higher education, dabbling in various careers, or settling down in a chosen vocation. As your second decade in life whirled by, you may have exchanged your first life role as dependent daughter with some mixture of roles such as hoyden, scholar, girlfriend, worker, explorer, or interdependent life partner. Then, before too many years passed, you may have chosen to start a family, ultimately adopting or turning down the role of mother.

If you opted for motherhood, whether as a single mother or as part of a long-term relationship, this seemingly simple decision then reconfigured your life. And whether your journey led you to become a wife, partner, career woman, stay-at-home mom, or some blend of these, the roles may have then *become your life*. As children grew, family expanded, and career developed, you may have lost yourself within the roles themselves. It may seem that every day brought yet another challenge that demanded more of you than you knew you had to give. But you gave, you accomplished, and you moved forward one step at a time. In all of this busyness of life, your twenties, thirties, forties, and even fifties may have whirled by in a blur.

Now whether you are on the brink of your fifties, sixties, or beyond, these blurred energies and experiences may be asking for attention. Those twenty, thirty, or forty-plus years that whirled past like a chronic monsoon may want to be noticed and honored. Indeed, these most beautiful—if daunting and challenging—years are what have made you the incredibly wonderful woman you are today. Whether difficult, fulfilling, joyful, incredibly demanding, or some mixture of all these, the roles, relationships, and ways of being you embraced in your past are a part of you. This awareness is a most beautiful and priceless possession, for it allows you to honor all that you are and all that you have done. This is the time to honor not just the good bits, not just the successes, but all of it—every hurt, sorrow, stumble, and fall. Every little piece. All of these riches and treasures of life are within you.

This is your time to reflect and consider both where you have been and what lies before you. Whether you had the opportunity to choose your life roles and relationships carefully or whether you unknowingly took what was imposed on you by others or happenstance, you can now breathe into these rich spaces of your life. Now is the time to wisely delve inside yourself and consider what has worked for you, what has not, and what you might like to do differently. Perhaps you are completely content with where you are in life, yet you may also crave change. It may be that you desire a slight shift here or there, or perhaps you are thirsty for something entirely new. Whatever you wish to be and do—whatever role and journey changes you envision—the gifts of reinvention await you. This, dear woman, can be a most spacious, reflective, and welcoming time in your life.

The History of Your Roles

As you begin to ponder reinventing your life roles, you might want to start by reflecting a bit more on your past. As you read the first part of this chapter, you may have become more aware of how busy you have been, how much you have given, and how many roles you have reflexively played. To honor as much of this as possible, you might want to write a letter to yourself—a letter of appreciation for all that you have accomplished. Perhaps this letter will, page by page, take you on a journey through each decade of your life. Written without judgment and with simple appreciation, this letter to yourself might be just what your soul needs to gain a bit of clarity and release.

To help you get started, below is a sample letter from a recent women's workshop. Let's imagine that this letter was written by a woman named Sarah, a woman who was looking at her past roles with growing awareness—and a mixture of sorrow, pride, and regret. As you read Sarah's letter, notice if you identify with certain aspects of her life.

Dear Soon-to-Be-Sixty Sarah,

Life hasn't been easy, has it? What a lot of living I've packed into these past fifty-nine years. Sometimes I feel as if I might explode with all the sadness, upheaval, pains, and crazy times I've experienced. Sure, there have been wonderful times, but it's the challenges that seem to stick with me the most. Maybe it's the regrets—not regrets about what I have done, but about the things I haven't done. I want to write about where I've been and the roles I've adopted.

Birth to Age 10: I don't remember too much. Our house was crazy. Dad was always gone and Mom was always angry. My older sister ignored me and my younger brother tormented me. School wasn't much better. I was somewhere in the middle of everything. I wasn't too smart or dumb. I wasn't particularly good at anything except being invisible.

I spent most of my first decade hiding in my room. I had a few friends at school who were quiet and invisible like me, but I was essentially a loner. I didn't want to compete. I didn't want to draw attention to myself. I wanted to blend in.

My roles: Invisible daughter. Solitary student. Fearful, timid friend.

Age 10 to Age 20: This part of my life was pretty much a dreary continuation of my first decade. Dad and Mom divorced and big sis left for college. Dad left and Mom became even angrier. It was up to me to keep a semblance of peace in the house—my mother and brother were constantly at it.

School and friendships were predictably mediocre. My friendships were more like crutches to avoid being alone. My first boyfriend was average. The loss of my virginity was quietly average. I wanted a fresh start, and I set my sights on college.

My roles: Peacemaker daughter. Average student. Fearful, grasping friend. Mediocre girl with a mediocre boyfriend. Young woman with a glimmer of aspiration.

Age 20 to Age 30: My twenties changed me. I moved two states away to go to college. Being away from home was rough, but not as rough as being at home. Money was tight. School was hard. Waiting tables gave me the money I needed, and it brought me out of my shell.

I wasn't at the top of my class at school, but I learned a lot. More than anything, I learned about myself and life. I learned how to open up to form friendships. I learned the ins and outs of being a roommate. I explored dating. I discovered the fun side of sex; it was far from mediocre. I discovered the playful, smart, fun side of me. I decided I wanted a career in nursing. I explored my options and selected the perfect nursing program. I felt like I had found my calling in life.

My roles: Good-enough college student. Hardworking waitress. Roommate. Caring friend. Playful, curious lover. Committed nursing student. Dedicated, passionate nurse.

Age 30 to Age 40: Nursing was the perfect fit for me. The work was hard and the hours were long—but I loved it. I enjoyed the friendships I formed at work. I dated a lot, but not seriously. I fell in love with cooking, my first real hobby. At thirty-three, I met the man who was to become my husband. We clicked on all levels and it seemed like life was bringing me everything I wanted. Shortly after I turned thirty-five, we married. I had my first child at thirty-six and our second child fifteen months later. Our third son arrived just shy of my thirty-ninth birthday.

Balancing home life and work life became too stressful. I had one foot in the nursing world and another at home—I never felt truly present in either place. After much discussion, I decided to leave nursing in favor of being a stay-at-home mother. It seemed like a good choice at the time, but I felt stifled.

My roles: Devoted nurse. Good friend. Aspiring cook. Passionate lover. Good wife. Hardworking, stay-at-home mother. Invisible woman.

Age 40 to Age 50: My forties disappeared; I don't know where they went. Somewhere between sleepless nights, colds and flus, homework, Little League games, two golden retrievers, loads of laundry, and making endless meals, I lost myself. At some point in all of this, I also lost my husband. As I was doing the laundry, I found a love note in my husband's pocket. It wasn't from me; it was from his secret lover. At forty-six, with three young boys, I couldn't decide if to stay or to leave.

My roles: Devoted and unfulfilled stay-at-home mother. Excellent cook. Good wife. Rage-filled wife. Betrayed wife. Lost woman.

Age 50 to Age 59: I tried the route of forgiveness but realized that some things can't be forgiven. By the time I turned fifty-three, what had become a vicious divorce finally resolved. I got the house and the kids. He got a new girlfriend. One-by-one, the boys left for college. I was left with an empty nest, friendships gone by the wayside, and ailing parents who lived 1,000 miles away. I refocused. By age fifty-five, I'd gotten up to speed and returned to nursing part-time. I felt out of place; so much had changed in my sixteen-year absence from nursing life. Now at fifty-nine, I make a vow to become un-lost.

My roles: Bitter ex-wife. Relieved divorcee. Proud mother. Empty nester. Frustrated daughter. Part-time, middle-aged nurse. Disconcerted, hopeful woman looking to reinvent herself.

And so, dear Self, here's to becoming un-lost. Here's to appreciating all the roles I embraced—the good and the not-so-good, the comfortable and the not-so-comfortable. Here's to patting myself on the back for trying so hard and growing so much. It's my goal to harvest the wisdom my life experiences have given me, using that wisdom to consciously make these next decades work for me.

With love and appreciation for all you have been and all you are to be,

Sarah

Sarah's contemplative, heartfelt letter gave her the opportunity to explore her history in an honest, clarifying way. Her letter, which took her several heart-wrenching drafts to complete, was both illuminating and cathartic. Indeed, a letter such as Sarah's can be helpful in letting you filter through some of your past memories and ways of being. The actual action of writing such a letter can move the psyche to release stored up thoughts, emotions, and energy.

Wisdom Tip 35: Write a "My Roles through Life" Letter to Yourself.

Create a safe, quiet space for writing to yourself. Allow your psyche to flow freely and without judgment as you write in your journal. As always, avoid the temptation to criticize your words or grammar—just write!

When your letter is completed, set it aside. After a space of time (be it a few hours or days later), read your letter with an open heart and open mind. When your process is complete, make notes about whatever thoughts and feelings arise.

Wisdom Tip 36: Nurture Appreciation for Your Life Roles.

When you are ready, sit quietly with yourself and re-read your letter. Allow the images of your roles—this history—to flow before you. The goal is simply to allow yourself to nonjudgmentally appreciate the roles you have held and carried. As your inner messages arise, let yourself appreciate them nonjudgmentally; let them inform you.

Feel free to re-write your letter a time or two more if your instinct tells you that it is important to deepen or continue your self-appreciation in this area. Strive to be free of self-judgment. When your work in this area feels complete, set it aside as a testament to your precious life journey.

Regrets and Gifts: The Lessons of Your Roles

One of the lovely aspects of maturation can be an increased interest in self-reflection. The later decades of life tend to offer more space and time for turning inward to look at one's interior world. This shift allows the opportunity for a heightened level of self-awareness. This may be the perfect time to get to know yourself intimately in ways that may have seemed unimportant or impossible in earlier years.

Of course, the woman who looks at you in the mirror today is an amalgamation of all that she has experienced and all that she has been. It can be easy to get stuck stewing on the past—shaming the self over bygone mistakes and unfulfilled dreams—and living with hurtful regret. There is no use in doing this; feelings such as shame and regret only cause more pain. Although life's hurts tend to get stuck in the psyche, you can learn to release them as they arise. You can set them free. By doing so, you free up all that space within your own being that was dark and cluttered. All the space that was formerly stagnant (held together by the sticky, toxic glue of negative, unproductive feelings and thoughts) will now be available to you for self-growth, love, and joy.

If you find yourself getting stuck in spaces filled with the likes of regret and shame, simply pause. Allow the thoughts and feelings to be present, and then consciously release them as if they are unwanted rocks or pebbles stuck in your mind or soul. Let them go. Do not judge yourself, your thoughts, or your feelings. Simply let them be present for a moment before you set them free. This may be very difficult for you to do at first, but it will become easier with practice. You are simply training your mind and body to work in a new direction; you are teaching it the power of releasing stuck or pent-up energy. You are teaching the mind that you'd rather use your energy to create joy. You are teaching your body that you don't want to hold on to negative energy—the very energy that can create tension and toxicity in your body.

As you practice this, you may feel a sense of grace descend upon you or move through you. This sense of grace may feel warm, soft, and enlivening. It may give you gentle chills. You may experience this grace as a sense of ease, release, and calm. The more you practice releasing stored up negative thoughts and bodily energy, the more you will feel grace living within you. This expansive sense of grace frees your being to expand into greater love and joy. This expansiveness will allow you to know a sense of self-love unlike anything you may have ever experienced. It will allow you to love, and be loved, in ways that are beyond the hurtful confines of negativity like shame and regret—the confines of fear.

Your letter to yourself might offer you the perfect opportunity to practice releasing negative thoughts and negative energy. Take a moment to re-read or re-imagine your letter, noticing any thoughts or feelings that bring up a constriction in your being. Notice any words or phrases that prompt a sense of negativity, whether it is regret, shame, guilt, or some other destructive feeling.

For example, in looking at Sarah's letter, you might have noticed that her letter is filled with a mixture of feelings such as confusion, pride, irritation, rage, sorrow, happiness, and regret. All of these feelings are normal and to be expected as a result of having experienced the joys and challenges of life. Yet holding onto the stuck, negative energy serves no positive purpose. The action of holding on to negativity only stores the destructive patterns (the negative energy) inside the self. Herein lies the perfect opportunity to create inner freedom. By seeking out each one of these stuck spots and releasing the stored energy, the self becomes more and more free. Of course, the release might not occur all at once, as certain emotions and thoughts may be more stuck than others, yet the patient act of releasing again and again can become a new and freeing pattern.

This following exercise can become a wonderful gift in your life. You can achieve freedom from your negative forces by consciously practicing the following steps:

1. Without judgment, notice the negative energy and thoughts when they arise. The unsettling energy arises first, yet the negative *thought* is often perceived first.

2. Immediately "breathe into" the thought and feeling without judgment as you create expansive space in your chest.

3. Breathe out powerfully, releasing the negative thought and energy with full force. You may wish to imagine a balloon popping as you release the stored energy out into the atmosphere where it scatters and floats away.

4. When negative energy thoughts and feelings return (as they surely will at some point) repeat this process without any self-judgment.

5. Be patient with yourself as you continue this practice over and over again; it may feel tiresome at first, yet you will come to honor and appreciate the results.

Practice this gentle exercise often, for it will allow you to detach from and release your stuck emotions and negative thoughts. The more you release negative forces, the lighter and more serene you will feel.

Your letter is powerful in another way, for it provides the perfect opportunity to notice the gifts of your roles. When you re-read or re-imagine your letter, notice any thoughts or feelings that feel expansive and light. Notice any words or phrases that create a sense of positivity; this may feel like happiness, delight, freedom, or some other uplifting sensation. You might not have paid attention to these positive feelings during your earlier readings of your letter; it can be human nature to give more attention to that which is hurtful and negative. But in this reading of your letter, notice all the pieces that give you any sense of deep *joy* or *delight*. Allow yourself to pause in these sections. Embrace any aspect—no matter how small—that feels energetically positive. Notice the roles that enriched you, gave you delight, and made you feel more whole. It is likely that these were the roles and experiences that were most meaningful to you—and those that felt most *right* to you. Allow yourself to notice the gifts within these experiences and roles.

As you prepare to enliven these next decades of your life, permit yourself to breathe into all that was a gift in your past; allow it to nourish you and propel you forward. This process will help you to create incredible inner freedom. As you seek out each space that holds positive energy, you give yourself permission to expand this energy. And as you learn to notice the positive thoughts and sensations—and then release them—your sense of grace and joy will expand.

Different in focus from the previous exercise, this next practice will allow you to notice and amplify the positive energies in your life. You will need to repeat this wonderful process again and again until it becomes second nature. In time, this exercise will become a precious gift in your life. By consciously practicing the following steps, you will enliven your inner sense of joy and grace:

1. Simply notice, without judgment, when positive energy and thoughts arise.
2. Immediately "breathe into" the thought and feeling as you envision creating open, expansive space in your chest.
3. Breathe out slowly, allowing the positive thought and energy to move through your body and then out of you. You might want to imagine joyful particles expanding and floating away like butterflies.
4. Every time you notice a positive thought or energy, repeat this process with an open heart.
5. If negative energy wants to move inward, release it.

This practice may feel unfamiliar and unnatural, yet the results will allow you to feel your natural joy and grace. *Notice that this practice can help you awaken and enliven your radiant, free-spirited self, the one that may have been quashed and left behind as you took on other roles in life. This childlike soul—so full of passion and joy—has been waiting for you all this time.*

Sarah's situation can help you deepen your awareness of this process. Indeed, Sarah was intent on moving into her sixties with free and positive energy. With a newfound sense that time was rushing by, Sarah wanted to "shake things up" quickly. Sarah liked the idea of using the letter she had written to herself as fuel to move forward. Using her letter as a guide, Sarah visualized each life stage and the roles she carried within each stage. When Sarah noticed a positive thought or feeling, something that gave her joy or pride, Sarah learned to breathe into that thought and feeling in a most expansive way. Then she would release the energy, imagining it floating through her and through the world. She devoted energetic time to appreciating the positive feelings that flooded her when she thought of her role as a loving mother. She also spent time noticing the positive energy she felt as she noticed herself as a playful lover, caring friend, committed nursing student, and devoted nurse. Sarah paused to notice the positive thoughts and feelings that were associated with her roles and experiences. She learned to breathe into these positive feelings and then release them with radiant warmth. Sarah allowed herself to nurture and expand the playful, passionate energy that had been minimized and forgotten, and she continued to notice and encourage all that felt positive to her.

As well, Sarah learned to give fleeting attention to her negative thoughts and feelings. Whenever negative energy arose, Sarah noticed that she felt "a stuck, dark knot inside." When Sarah felt this knot (whether it held anger, fear, shame, or guilt), she consciously breathed into the negative energy and then she released it. Although it seemed counter-intuitive to her at first, Sarah found incredible release from this process. At the same time, Sarah discovered that her feelings of sorrow and regret often returned, almost as if the source of them was endless. She noted that her sense of regret felt particularly strong; it seemed "sticky" and depressing. Indeed, heavy bricks of regret seemed to block Sarah's forward movement; however, Sarah persisted in her practice of releasing the negative forces that had built up inside her year after year. Every time a negative energy and thought arose, she reminded herself to breathe into it fully and then release it. Sarah was, over time, able to release many of her stored up resentments from childhood and beyond.

As an example, Sarah released the sorrows and resentments she held for her role as a frightened, invisible child. She released a role that had unconsciously remained with her—the lingering role of feeling mediocre and believing she deserved a mediocre life. Sarah also discovered that she had a silent fear that she was "too old" to return to her beloved role as a nurse. She released this deep-seated fear and chose to embrace a new role—that of a seasoned woman who had much to offer in the form of dedicated service, knowledge, and life experience.

Now and again, Sarah revisited the letter she had written to herself. She learned to delight in the process, for the letter became symbolic of her courage and willpower. If she felt a new or recurring negative pull from any aspect of the letter, she simply took it as an indication that some piece of negative energy had welled up and needed to be released. So she would free the energy and move on. In this way, Sarah found release from anger over her marriage. She was able to cleanse herself from the negative residue of her husband's betrayal. With her children gone, Sarah began volunteering at a food kitchen, using her love for cooking to help feed others. She began dating and rejuvenated her role of passionate lover, a role she had left by the wayside. Sarah was also able to find healing that allowed her to embrace a compassionate role as her elderly parents' caring daughter.

Sarah's process was not simple or easy, but it ultimately released the stuck energy that had held her back. Through the process of seeing the gifts within each role (and releasing any negative thoughts and feelings), Sarah found freedom. All of this allowed Sarah to ultimately reinvent herself from the inside out. She used her wisdom to create a joyful life that worked for her—a life filled with meaning and promise. Sarah found that her life hadn't ended in her fifties; *it had just begun.*

Sarah's process of letting go and expanding is surely available to you. Nothing need hold you back from entering the next phase of your life filled with positive energy; nothing can stop you from releasing the contaminants that are inside of you. (Common contaminants include shame, regret, and guilt, but many others may arise.) Trust that, like Sarah, you can utilize your history to create an incredible future. Regular use of two simple tools can free your energy to embark on new journeys: remember to *notice and release* any negative energy (anything that does not serve you), and strive to *notice and feel* the flow of all positive energy. Through this process, you will embrace the wisdom you have earned, and its radiance will help you better envision and enliven this next wondrous phase of your life.

Reinventing Your Roles with a Wise Heart

Reinventing oneself and one's roles isn't always easy. In fact, given that people tend to resist change with tremendous energy, self-reinvention can feel extremely painful. On a positive note, you will find that change needn't be excruciating. It's simply that we are often wired to fear change as if it is an enemy. As a result, we get stuck in life and avoid the natural movement that would allow us to evolve more fully, keeping us caught in the same patterns, roles, and ways of being that make us feel strangled and unfulfilled. To understand this concept better, let's take a look at Emma, who, at age sixty-three, discovered that she was fed up with a few key roles she had adopted in life.

Emma found herself staring at her sixty-fourth birthday on her calendar as if it were a make-or-break date. She wanted change (and believed that she *needed* change) before another year ticked by; however, Emma was terrified of what the future might look like if she shifted her life. The decision she contemplated—leaving her marriage of nearly thirty years—had myriad ramifications. In hindsight, Emma realized that she had only half-enjoyed the past three decades with her husband. Drawn to him through the magnet of mutual interests and life goals, Emma and her spouse had each achieved tremendous financial success. Neither Emma nor her husband, Aaron, wanted a family. And so, without children to distract them, they each forged lucrative businesses that filled their days.

Emma appreciated Aaron's intense drive and ambition; these traits seemed to meld with her own life goals. Yet Emma also noticed an interesting tendency in Aaron; the more success he achieved, the harder he worked to surpass his own goals. Over time, Aaron lost interest in connecting with Emma sexually. The emotional intimacy they once had also began to fade. When Emma tried to talk with Aaron about her concerns, Aaron would say she was being "too sensitive" and that "everything would work out fine." However, one project after another took Aaron's full attention. As the years passed by, the distance between them continued to grow. Emotional and sexual disconnection became their customary normal. Feeling pushed aside, Emma focused on her own business and began to invest more time into cultivating friendships with like-minded women. These friendships gave Emma some of the emotional support and connection she longed for from Aaron.

Emma continued to plod along, enjoying her business, occasional travels with Aaron, and her deep connection to her girlfriends. All the while, a part of her interior world seemed to die away. Emma knew in her heart that she was not in an emotionally fulfilling relationship, but she accepted it as "good enough." After all, she had all the financial stability and material trappings a person would want. When her frustrations built up, Emma would share her discontent with her husband; each time, he shrugged off her concerns as a "late-life midlife crisis." Her husband repeatedly refused marital therapy, so Emma sought out an individual therapist of her own. In addition, Emma found herself increasingly sharing her dissatisfaction with her girlfriends instead of her husband. In weekly "venting lunches," the women each aired complaints and vented their anger, but nothing was ever resolved. Every woman in the group was afraid of making a shift, anxiously evading the much-coveted, but highly feared, positive change. And so, each passing month brought more distance between Emma and her husband.

Frustrated and angry, Emma found a different way to have her emotional and sexual needs met; she opted to find fulfillment through an extramarital affair. In this secretive relationship, Emma found the passion she had been craving. She delighted in the secrecy, sex, and connection she shared with her new man. At sixty-four, Emma felt as if she were in the prime of her life—she felt more playful and sexual than she had ever been. In the role of desired paramour, Emma felt beautiful, young, and free. Her new sweetheart showered her with affection, secret gifts, and adoration. Emma was filled with newfound happiness—until fate had its way.

One morning, as she rushed out the door to make a morning appointment across town, Emma accidentally left her phone at home. She realized her mistake a few hours later. Fear welled up inside her when she realized her phone was not in her purse or her car. Worried that she might have left the phone where her husband might see it, Emma worked out the possible scenarios on her way home. If a phone call or text message had uncovered the affair, she decided to face it openly. Pressing her anxiety aside, Emma came to the same conclusion she had before: Aaron had emotionally abandoned her, and this forced her to seek sexual and emotional connection elsewhere. Emma's fears came to life when she walked in the front door to her see her husband's scowling, angry face. Indeed, her lover had texted her several times, and her husband had seen the texts. Emma stood her ground with quiet determination as Aaron fumed and ranted. Aaron wanted the affair to stop immediately; Emma did not.

Uncertain about how to proceed with her life, Emma came to see me. As I listened to her talk about the past thirty years of her life, I could tell that lines of resentful resignation had been etched into Emma's heart. Emma noted, "He doesn't know how to love anything but money and pride. At first he was furious with me about the affair, but I didn't let him bully me. Yes, I had a sexual affair for a few months, but he had a thirty-year affair with his business and his material possessions. There was always another deal, another meeting, and more money to be made. Enough was never enough for him—unless it had to do with being close to me. In that case, even a little bit was too much."

Emma's resentment and anger filled the room. "We just started marriage therapy," she continued. "It was his idea. And believe it or not, he started individual therapy as well. After all this time, now he wants to save the marriage. Now he wants to make it work. But you know what? I don't know if I do. I don't trust him. I think he'll just do this for a few months, maybe even a year, and then go back to the way he was. If I buy into this, I'll have wasted another year of my life. I am tired of wasting my years."

"Emma," I said, "I understand how angry you are at your husband; that makes perfect sense. I am also wondering if there's something more to your anger—if there's something or someone else you are angry at."

"What do you mean?" Emma questioned.

I responded, "I wonder if, perhaps, you are also angry at yourself."

Emma reached for tissues to dab the tears that welled up in her eyes. "Yes, I am. I am mad at myself. I am mad that I let my life slip away. In fact, I'm furious with myself for putting up with all of this for so long. I knew I wasn't happy, but I didn't do anything about it. I kept hoping things would change, even when it was clear they were getting steadily worse. In the end, I am mad at him for being so self-obsessed. External success has been everything to him. Our success as a couple—and my happiness—were not important at all. I didn't want to acknowledge this. Now that I do, I'm very angry at myself for not leaving sooner. It's what I should have done twenty-five years ago."

Emma's pain was palpable. She was angry at her husband for his self-obsession, and she was angry with herself for her own obsession with avoiding the truth she knew inside. But even with her growing awareness, it was difficult for Emma to choose her course. She had built a home with her husband for three decades. She was comfortable in life—comfortable with her material world, her friendships, and the day-to-day pattern of her life. Was the search for a different life and a new mate worth unsettling every aspect of her world? It was the same choice she had silently noticed decades earlier, yet her life was even more cemented now.

Emma knew a divorce would create intense disruptions on many levels. She knew that she wouldn't want to stay in their house; she felt drawn to create a new home of her own. As well, most of Emma's friends were married to husbands who liked and respected Aaron. Emma knew that a divorce would strain, and even end, some of these friendships. Emma was aware that even the daily pace of her life would change dramatically if she left;

there would be no extra body in the house with whom to share meals, a bed, and morning banter. Emma didn't relish the role of being single and in her mid-sixties, but neither did she relish the role of being an unhappy, unfulfilled wife. Of course, I couldn't tell Emma what course to take, I could only help her envision the roles and the courses—the possibilities—that were open to her. One or more of these possibilities might lead to the future she longed to create; in the end, the choice would be Emma's. Yet to make a wise decision, Emma needed to process and release her anger. And in order to move forward, Emma needed to leave resentment behind—resentment at herself and at her husband—for what had happened in the past.

To find her answer, Emma strove to release her anger and resentment. She worked diligently at imagining the possibilities that could bring her joy and inner peace. Using a wise blend of imagination and self-honesty, Emma played with the possibilities. In time, Emma pared down her imaginings to a select few. She envisioned remaining in the marriage as planned—coming to a place of firm acceptance of what she had chosen. She also pondered the idea of staying for one more year—long enough to see if her husband's promised changes would take hold. As another option, Emma considered the idea of remaining in the marriage but demanding that her husband agree that she could have affairs as she pleased. However, Emma's thoughts turned, most frequently, to the idea of being a single woman exploring herself and eventually opening up to find a loving mate. Emma pondered this option repeatedly. The more she explored the idea, the more Emma felt that it was the right choice. Although she knew the road wouldn't be easy, Emma came to peace with the idea of filing for divorce, purchasing her own home, and setting up a fresh, single life.

Emma realized that it ultimately didn't matter whether the new "single woman" life she envisioned would lead to the romantic relationship of her dreams. Emma discovered that she simply wanted and needed so much more from life than what she had. She was no longer willing to settle for "good enough." As her future opened up before her, new role options populated her mind. Almost magnetized by her shift in attitude, opportunities came toward Emma. From an offer for a new business partnership to a volunteer position mentoring young women, Emma found that she was in demand. There came a time that she knew, in her heart, that she was ready to move forward. Emma listened to her inner voice and decided to part ways with her husband. In a conscious, graceful way, she ultimately created the life she had craved for so many years.

Like Emma, you can use your heart and your wisdom to consider the roles and the journey that is just right for you. Your shifts do not need to be dramatic. Marriages and friendships need not go by the wayside. In fact, your personal relationships may be enhanced by your internal changes. What is most important is that you listen to the beat of your own heart and soul.

Notice the areas where you are constrained, and focus on healing and curing them. Notice the areas where you feel lush and fluid, and focus on creating more of that sacred energy. You will find that your future holds tremendous possibilities, but take note that you may tend to narrow your focus if you feel fearful. As you contemplate change, you might notice that the least unsettling options often *appear* to be better choices, as the more challenging and upending options tend to be a bit scarier. As you proceed with an open, nonjudgmental spirit, clarity will come. There is no singular "right" way to approach such deeply personal issues. What matters most is that you pause to consider what is right for you—for your beliefs, your soul, and your overall well-being. When you approach your life in this thoughtful and wise manner, doors will open and you will find your way—ever so gracefully, powerfully, and joyfully.

Redefining Your Relationships

Many of our relationships in life form as a result of natural, chance intersections. We do not choose what are often the most formative relationships of our lives, for we are "given" both our parents and our siblings. Even our friendships are often the result of chance connections during school, social events, or at work. If we are lucky, we might feel an instant "click" with a new acquaintance. This fledging relationship might develop over time with a true intimacy built on trust and shared hopes, joys, and challenges. As a result, such a relationship often becomes a deep friendship that can withstand the tests of time.

In many cases, however, what we call friendships might be more aptly termed acquaintances. These are the connections that develop when we simply gravitate to someone who shares a common interest or makes us feel less alone in a crowd. What differentiates true friendships from acquaintances is the level of trusting, intimate, and honest connection. Of course, there are varying levels and degrees within these types of relationships. Although each type of relationship has its place, it can be helpful to differentiate between them for many reasons. Such distinctions will help you understand the nature of your relationships—why some feel safer and more "real" and why others might leave you feeling uneasy or disconnected.

As you relax into this precious stage in your life, it is natural that you may be more aware of the relationships that feel positive and those that do not. Some wonderful relationships may have waned while others may have become static or toxic. Indeed, the concept of a relationship can shift and even take on an entirely new meaning as a person matures. This is a normal and natural part of the aging process. Having left behind the most distracting days of your life, these later decades may crystallize that which is dearest to you. This crystallization process may leave you noticing and redefining your relationships. This is your opportunity to pause to notice what you *want* from your relationships and what you want *to give* to your relationships. Now is your time to breathe into those relationships that you want to nurture. This is your opportunity to recreate relationships in a way that allows you and your loved ones to thrive. It may even be the time to set yourself free from relationships that are impossible to heal and have caused you to suffer. This stage of your life gives you the privilege and freedom of addressing all of your relationships with graceful wisdom.

Pause to notice the relationships in your life. If it is helpful, write out a list of your relationships—include family members, friendships, and acquaintances. Next to each person's name, make a note of the relationship type and quality as you see it. For example, you might note, "Elaine: treasured best friend," "Sam: steadfast running partner," "Kevin: devoted eldest son, "Kit: precious granddaughter," or "Will: difficult older brother." The purpose of such a list is not to judge the individuals or the relationships, but to determine the nature and quality of them with as much personal objectivity as possible.

Through this lens, you can evaluate how or if you want to shift any of your relationships. There may be some that you want to leave unchanged. Others may stand out as being ones to which you wish to devote more time and energy. Some may call out for attention in a way that may be healing. There may be a few relationships that you wish to loosen or discontinue altogether. As well, some relationships may simply ask for you to refocus and redefine the relationship as you see it now—to make shifts in your own psyche to come to peaceful terms with the relationship.

Once your list is complete, notice what you would like to give to each relationship. Make note of those that you want to nurture, enliven, or heal. Notice those that you wish to alter or redefine. Take note of those that you wish to accept with peace and those that you wish to release. For those relationships that are calling out for change, allow yourself to make a few specific, actionable ideas next to each name. For example, you may have written, "Mimi: destructive, passive-aggressive sister who calls me every day to complain." If you want to redefine this relationship and create a shift, you might write, "Mimi: troubled sister. I no longer want to have her disturbing energy in my life every day. I will set strong boundaries and talk with her for only ten minutes once a week." As another example, you may have noted, "Anne: longtime, cherished friend with whom I rarely connect." Next to Anne's name, you might note, "Anne: cherished childhood friend with whom I will connect on a weekly basis. I will reach out to set up coffee dates and hiking outings."

As you move through each relationship, your heart and your inner wisdom will guide you on the right path. This evaluative process is not necessarily easy, but it can be incredibly rewarding and healing. Time is precious and rarer with each passing moment; this truly is the time in your life to reflect on what you want. By giving your time and energy to the relationships that you value most, you are giving yourself one of the greatest gifts in life.

Understanding, Adapting, and Balancing Natural Changes in Key Relationships

Shifts in key relationships are often inherently difficult, yet a lack of understanding and awareness can make natural and necessary changes all the more challenging. This era of your life may certainly bring an interesting twist to many of the relationships in your life that were once fairly static. Maturing women face a host of new relationship dynamics as parents decline, partners age, and adult children spread their wings. By taking an honest, open look at the key relationships in your life, you will become more familiar with the dynamics of each relationship.

Although every relationship has its own unique dynamics, certain foundational factors tend to permeate all relationships. Some dynamics are more pronounced in certain relationship categories, such as those encountered with aging parents and adult children. You will feel more confident as you better understand and appreciate the nuances of these dynamics. With increased self-awareness and useable tips, you will feel more adept at gracefully and powerfully managing even the most difficult relationship issues.

This era of your life may have you laughing or shaking your head over the impact of your relationships and the patterns within them. You might notice that certain negative patterns from your own childhood persist in your relationships today. You might have purposefully shaken off old, unhealthy dynamics and created healthy ones that work for you. You may have always had rather healthy relationships and are looking only to refine and enliven those relationships. Wherever you are in this spectrum, know that you have the power to understand and create the dynamics that will make these next decades all the more beautiful.

In my work as a psychologist, I have discovered that the key factors permeating human relationships include *need, ability, desire, availability, willingness,* and *commitment.* These foundational blocks are the basis for nearly every relationship in life. A few examples will help you better understand these key factors. Using the parent-child relationship as an illustration, it can be fairly easy to see the "need" factor. The parent often feels the *need* to have a child, and the dependent child certainly *needs* the parent. The "ability" factor is clearly significant, for certain *abilities* are required of a healthy parent. As to the "desire" factor, it is important that parents have a deep *desire* to create and raise a child. When desire is present, the heart (the emotional connection) is involved. "Availability" is a vital factor, for emotional, mental, and physical *availability* are all key to a healthy relationship. The healthiest parent-child relationships are formed when the parents are *available* to the child in all three realms—emotionally, mentally, and physically. "Willingness" is another key factor, for the other factors are meaningless if an individual is not *willing* to act on the need, ability, desire, and availability factors. In the parent-child relationship, a parent can certainly have the need, ability, desire, and availability to have and raise a child, but if the parent does not have the *willingness* to follow through, the child will assuredly suffer.

Of course, the "commitment" factor is the absolute crowning jewel of these factors. Without *commitment,* no relationship—even those where all of the other factors are present—will be optimized.

In the parent-child relationship, it is clearly the parents who must be *committed* to the process. As with other relationships, strong parent-child connections tend to result when the six factors of need, ability, desire, availability, and willingness are pressed into concerted action.

Once you understand the importance of these factors across your various relationships, you will be able to more clearly examine why some of your relationships are more fulfilling and satisfying than others. You will better understand why some of your relationships go awry. Simply look at the six key factors—need, ability, desire, availability, willingness, and commitment—to see what is missing or out of balance. By utilizing this lens as you look at the relationships in your life, you will feel enlightened and empowered. In certain relationships you will be able to make easy, positive adjustments, yet some may be more difficult to shift. When you're equipped with wise awareness, patience, and a healthy dose of laughter, you'll be able to manage your relationships with greater understanding, acceptance, and grace.

Of course, some relationships are more intimate and connective in nature than others. Beyond the six key relationship factors lie other elements—such as strong affection, mutual interests, emotional intimacy, and romantic love—that have the power to create an even more profound bond. When elements such as these are present in addition to the six key factors, the resulting relationship can rise to the level of a wondrous, inimitable friendship. Relationships of this kind can be the greatest jewels and joys in one's life.

Thank you for having the courage to delve ever deeper into your life. You may now find that you know and appreciate yourself quite a bit more. You may have greater awareness of your life roles and relationships—what they have been, where they are now, and where you'd like them to be. Although the process of increasing self-awareness is often uncomfortable and even scary, the rewards are vast. In truth, there is no gift quite as precious in life as coming to learn and love all of who you are. It is from the vantage point of honest self-awareness that you can look in the mirror and say, "I love you deeply and truly. I love all of you. I love your wrinkles and your willing smile. I love your patience and the wisdom you've earned. I love that you've learned from your mistakes; they've taught you much of what you know. I love that you've embraced your triumphs and successes; they have given you great joy. You are tough. You are strong. You are courageous. You are resilient. You are beautiful."

CHAPTER 5

Embracing Changes in Relationships and Roles

*Y*our journey of self-reflection may leave you wondering and even pensive. As you evaluate your life as it is, it's only natural that you feel the stirring winds of change. All of this is normal and to be expected for a woman venturing forward with an open heart and a thoughtful, open mind. Indeed, change comes whether we want it or not. Our power lies in how we face the changes that necessarily come as part of life. Do you let worrisome fear or complacency hold you in place? Or do you venture forward with curiosity, wisdom, and an attitude of loving flexibility? Choose the path that is right for you; let your heart be your guide. When you act from a place of love, compassion, wisdom, and integrity, the important pieces tend to fall into place. The ribbon of life becomes all the more beautiful when you consciously take part in the process.

You now have the opportunity to more fully explore and embrace the changing relationships and roles in your life. So many changes—some incredibly delightful and some very challenging—surface during the later years of womanhood. When prepared with a bouquet of humor, thoughtful kindness, and gentle wisdom, even the most difficult changes can be faced with grace. You will make some missteps along the way (now and again we all do), yet that is life. If you stumble, find the lesson to be learned and smile. Womanhood is not about being perfect; it's about learning how to navigate life's difficulties and imperfect moments with courage and compassion. This is grace. This is the essence of womanhood in action.

Wisdom for Empty Nesters

Whether you had your children early or late in life, it's likely that your child-rearing years were consumed with tasks oriented toward loving, educating, and generally caring for your progeny. A woman may find that she lost her identity in the varied roles of motherhood that range from cook, nurse, and advocate to teacher, guide, and friend. Stay-at-home mothers (who often do not have other identities such as employee, boss, or business owner) often suffer the most when their young adult children prepare to leave home.

On one hand, you may be looking at your empty-nest years with enthusiastic delight, and on the other you may fear the empty spaces that were once occupied by your child's needs, desires, and energy. It's easy to say, "Don't worry about it! Your life will expand when your children are gone—you'll have so much free time. You'll be able to do anything you please!" Indeed, such sentiments are true, but they often seem like empty platitudes to the mother who faces the loss. It is in this space of loss and emptiness that wisdom waits for you.

Wisdom Tip 37: Allow Yourself to Feel Your Empty Nest Feelings.

As you look at your soon-to-be-empty or already empty nest, imagine the space with an open heart. Imagine what it will (or does) feel like without your child's presence. Allow yourself to experience and embrace the emotions that arise—whether they are sadness, anger, joy, or fear. Let each one arise in turn, allowing yourself to notice and breathe into the richness of your experience.

Of course, this process might not be painless, but it is real. In allowing yourself to experience your emotions, you will ultimately set them free to move out of you. You may need to repeat this process many times. You may want to cry, laugh, or throw an anger tantrum. Whatever you feel, allow yourself to experience it and embrace it. It's that simple. Notice it, feel it, and let it go.

When it was time for my first son to leave for college, we took the 550-mile journey by car. As I waited in the busy airport for my solo return trip home, I began to sob quietly in the midst of the busy airport. I let myself feel my pain and sorrow. With still-wet eyes, I boarded the plane a few minutes later.

The woman in front of me turned and said, "I can see you are sad. Are you okay?"

I smiled half-heartedly and replied, "My son has been at my side for nineteen years. Today, I'm leaving him at college. It hurts so much."

This loving woman reached out to pat my shoulder as she said, "I went through that a few years back. I cried like a baby for a few weeks straight. It will get better in time."

We shared a smile and the warmth of knowing that we were not alone—and that everything would be okay. Indeed, when it's time for a child to leave the nest, there is joy in knowing that we played a part in helping prepare the child to fly.

Wisdom Tip 38: Get to Know Your Empty Nest Fears.

So much of the empty-nest syndrome is built on fear. For example, empty-nesters often tell me that they fear having too much free time. They fear the loss of the endless to-do lists that were a natural part of child rearing. Empty-nesters often fear feeling purposeless, as if being a mother were their one and only calling in life. Some empty nesters fear a loss of connection with their child, a fear that the child will ultimately move and settle down in a different area. As well, empty nesters often worry that, without a child or children in the home, the marriage will change, suffer, or expose itself as a hollow relationship bound only by child-rearing.

All or some of these fears may be valid in some way or another. Yet the only way of exposing the fears for whatever they may be is to become familiar with the fears—to unearth them and inspect them. Once you acknowledge and understand the specific fears, you can embrace them and effect change.

For example, if a woman fears that her life will be without purpose without a child to raise, that fear could actually be true. Indeed, she could choose to remain confined in the role of paralyzed empty-nester, hovering over the young adult child or forever mourning the child's absence. Or she could choose to move through this blockage and fear to actively create new life purposes. Once change is envisioned and specific steps to effect change are outlined, all that is required is the desire and energy to make the changes come to life.

As you get to know and explore each empty-nester fear, you will find that each fear can be dismantled and worked through in this same way. The changes inherent in an empty nest may certainly be challenging and scary, but they need not be immobilizing. An empty nest can, indeed, have incredible spaciousness that waits to be filled and enjoyed.

Wisdom Tip 39: Move Forward by Making Plans and Letting Go.

Nothing makes letting go quite as easy as having new plans in the works. As you prepare to let go of your young adult children, make plans for reconnection. Having a date or two set on the calendar can give you the reassurance and hope you need to move forward with joy. When a child leaves for college or a job across the country, it can feel very affirming to know that tickets have already been purchased for holiday or birthday visits. If in-person visits are not possible given finances and distance, create weekly phone check-ins. Knowing the planned date of the next connection can help dissipate the lonely feelings of disconnection.

Remember that it's important to balance your desire for contact with your adult child's need for independence and autonomy. As one mother explained, "At first I wanted to call my daughter every night. I had to force myself not to text her every few hours. I had to learn to breathe through those urges in order to allow her to build her own friendships and college life. The first few weeks were terribly hard on me, but when she did call it felt wonderful to listen to her stories and hear enthusiasm in her voice. It made me feel good knowing that she felt secure enough to expand into her new life."

Wisdom Tip 40: Create Understandings and Maintain Good Boundaries to Foster Independence.

Once your adult child leaves the nest, remember that you are largely off duty. Although your child may still be dependent on you for tuition or rent subsidies, much of the child's daily life is now out of your control. This new era comes with both benefits and losses—both of which are best faced with clear understandings and solid boundaries.

It can be easy to get into the role of helicopter parent; the best way to avoid this pitfall is to create clear expectations and understandings for behaviors. Whether grades, part-time work, finances, substance use, or partying are issues of concern, set clear expectations and make sure the expectations are understood. Then use healthy boundaries to stick to whatever agreements have been made. This simple and straightforward approach will allow your adult child to develop healthy autonomy and self-responsibility. As well, you will benefit from knowing that you are completing your parenting duties in a strong and healthy way.

As an example, a couple I worked with set clear boundaries for their college-bound son about their expectations regarding grades and finances. Although their son kept his grades in the right range, he often called to get additional funds due to overspending. The couple could financially afford the requests for extra money, but they knew it was important for their son to manage his funds properly. And so, after the third month of sending extra funds, they restated the financial boundaries with kindness and clarity. Although their son was miffed at them for a few days, he ultimately apologized and obtained an on-campus job that afforded him the extra spending money he wanted. It is through such actions that parents can continue to build an adult child's sense of self-respect and personal responsibility.

Wisdom Tip 41: Breathe and Prepare for Change.

Your life will never be the same as it was when you were actively parenting. When you feel at a loss in your new role, pause to breathe. Continue to notice that the loss of your role as active parent will continue to lessen. This is a normal and necessary aspect of life. Your child may return to the nest, but the child who returns will be different—and so will you.

One of my clients described her daughter's unexpected transformation during a summer internship in a large city. She noted, "When my daughter left home, she had a boyfriend, light-brown hair, and a preppy sort of style. When she returned a few months later, she had a girlfriend, dyed-green hair, and three tattoos. It was a shock, but I am working to embrace it all. I realize that I want her to be herself—even if it means that she's someone else entirely the next time she comes home."

Of course, an adult child's changes can be unsettling. As long as they are not harmful to the self or others, such changes are a natural part of maturation. Strive to not be frightened of these changes— strive to embrace this new era with joy and delight. As you make space for your adult child's choices and newfound autonomy, you will also be making space in your own heart for freedom and new flights of your own.

Taking Care When Adult Children Return Home

Just when you get used to your freedom—to filling the empty nest with new activities and friends—your adult child may want or need to return home. Life has a way of bringing shifts like this, almost as if life wants to challenge our patience. In fact, given the economic climate in the world, an increasing number of adult children find it necessary or comfortable to return home for a short or extended period of time. Some mothers unconsciously assume that their child's return will be easy and that things will be much the same as when the child was younger; however, this is rarely the case as the adult child can be more independent and space-taking in nature. Some parents fear setting ground rules, yet clear agreements will support respectful behavior and family harmony. There's no particular right or wrong way to handle an adult child's return, yet a few basic guidelines can make the transition easier for everyone.

Wisdom Tip 42: Create House Rules to Facilitate Harmony.

Although it may seem bothersome to create household agreements for adult children, a simple, clear outline can save a great deal of resentment and negativity. In developing your personalized agreement, it's important that you know what is and is not important for you to address. Simple house rules can include the following:

1. How long the adult child will stay in the home;
2. How much the child will contribute in rent and toward utilities;
3. Use of family items, such as vehicles, etc.;
4. Contributions to insurance for use of vehicles, etc.;
5. Expectations regarding guests and pets;
6. Expectations regarding alcohol and substance use;
7. Expectations regarding food use and contribution to food costs;
8. Expectations for adult child's employment or employment pursuit;
9. Expectations for contributions to household tasks (kitchen duties, general cleaning, trash duties, etc.);
10. Expectations for general cleanliness standards (bedroom, kitchen, etc.);
11. Expectations for involvement in family activities (family parties, religious activities, etc.);
12. Agreement regarding moving out, should the adult child be unwilling to honor any part of the mutual agreement.

After feeling like an unwanted guest in her own home, one client in her sixties found herself working out an agreement with her adult son and his girlfriend several months after they had moved in. Unused to setting clear boundaries, it was challenging for her to create and institute the agreement. Yet a few weeks after the house rules were defined, she was proud of her efforts and the positive results.

Wisdom Tip 43: Hold Fast to Agreements as You Let Go of Minor Issues.

Once you have established your house rules and agreements have been made, be firm. Like young children, some returning adult children test a parent's limits. Hold fast and true, knowing that you created the agreement to protect your sanity and your relationships.

Your job at this stage is to remain steadfast in ensuring that your adult child handles his or her responsibilities with respect. When respectful behavior is the norm, you can allow yourself to let go. A mutually respectful relationship will allow your adult child to move forward in an autonomous way, feeling free of guilt or embarrassment for returning home. The clear and firm boundaries you have taken the time to set will allow you to feel great about yourself and your new relationship with your child.

As one sixty-two-year-old mother noted, "I had mixed feelings when my daughter returned home after she split up with her fiancé. I wanted her to feel welcome and safe, but she created more drama than she did in high school. One day she surprised us by bringing home a puppy, and then she wanted to bring a new boyfriend into our home. My husband and I were starting to bicker with all the tension, so we had to be firm with her. We set rules on the important things like the puppy, the boyfriend, and her responsibilities. My husband and I decided —as a team—to overlook the smaller stuff (like the way she kept her bathroom and her habit of leaving the television on). When she saw that we were going to be firm and not get drawn into her unnecessary drama, her own attitude shifted."

Such shifts in attitude and behavior can create an environment that feels relaxing, safe, and respectful for everyone.

Wisdom Tip 44: Avoid the Pitfalls of Shaming, Blaming, and Guilt-Tripping.

An adult child often feels disappointed or ashamed by the need to return home. Our independence-oriented culture often stigmatizes adult children who return to live with their parents. An underlying sense of shame can erode an adult child's sense of self-esteem and self-respect.

Given this truth, it's important to support your adult child's return home in a proactive and loving way. This doesn't mean that you give into the adult child's demands or pay his or her way. In fact, the opposite is true. Your adult child will feel more valuable when you set clear expectations in a loving, non-shaming way. However, if you give something to your child (whether it is financial, material, or emotional support), do so without attaching any strings. If your attitude becomes blaming, shaming, or guilt-inducing, both you and your adult child will suffer. Use your inner wisdom to support your adult child's ongoing journey in a way that is firm, kind, and respectful.

One client, just on the verge of turning sixty, welcomed her hardworking son's return after his graduation from college. The last of her three children, the pair had always had a good relationship. Her son hadn't yet been able to find a position in his chosen career, but he pressed forward with his job search. Seeing his contributions to home life and his dedication to the temporary job he had taken, she gave him money to buy a sturdy used car. However, as happens, the two had a heated disagreement over a minor issue.

My client's temper flared, and she told her son, "You are so ungrateful. I gave you money for a car, and you can't even run an errand for me!"

The son wisely told my client, "Mom, don't give me anything if there are strings attached. It's not good for either of us."

My client humbly shared this story with me. Indeed, she had learned from her own son the importance of giving gifts—be they gifts of time, money, material items, or something else—without expectations or conditions attached.

The Ins and Outs of Married/ Partnered Children and Grandchildren

As families grow and expand, unhealthy patterns and behaviors can become more pronounced. Even the healthiest of families can face times of stress and strain as a result of the changes experienced in this new phase of life. As adult children choose partners and begin to have families of their own, a host of both wonderful and challenging issues can arise. As with most aspects of life, the more prepared a woman is to face the changes, the easier the changes will be. Although certain tips will be helpful in embracing this new phase, personal awareness is always a critical component. In truth, it is the wisdom and self-assurance that come with increased selfawareness and understanding that make every difference in family dynamics.

Many women naturally delight in the thought of having a new son- or daughter-in-law. Some women also look forward to the idea of having a brood of grandchildren to nurture and love. Indeed, some women begin to crave having grandchildren even before their own children have matured. Other women are less inclined to want an influx of new family members—whether they are children or adults. As with most such arenas of life, there is no right or wrong way to approach this era of life. What is most critical is that you know what is right and true for you. Once you come to terms with your personal preferences, you will be able to honor the areas you want to open and expand. You will also be able to own the resistance you may have in certain realms. Whatever your preferences may be, you will ultimately be able to set boundaries that are clear and consistent. All of this will allow you to embrace your adult children, their partners, their little ones, and extended family with grace and ease.

Wisdom Tip 45: Institute and Maintain Healthy Boundaries.

If you didn't have strong, clear boundaries with your child in earlier years, it may be difficult for the child to accept your new, healthy boundaries. However, all you need do is be firm and consistent with your boundaries; your child will eventually get the message that "Mom is no longer a pushover."

As your adult child brings a partner into your life, take the time to discuss boundaries with your child. Boundaries may include limitations on financial assistance or other demands. As adult children often return home for holidays and other events, family policies regarding pets, sleeping arrangements, expected behavior, and substance use are some common topics that benefit from open and honest discussion. As well, boundaries may need to be set for extended family members, particularly if some relatives have not cultivated healthy boundaries of their own.

When it comes to grandchildren, clear and simple boundaries for all parties will make life much easier. From helping with childcare to having boundaries regarding behavior in your home, everyone will feel more relaxed if expectations are simple, consistent, and straightforward.

Wisdom Tip 46: Know the Type of Relationships You Want and Accept the Type of Relationships Others Want.

Many relationships suffer when the parties have different needs and goals. As you expand your family to include your adult child's partner, children, and extended family, it's up to you to know what type of relationships you would like to have with each person. Some women are terrifically excited to embrace new relatives, and others feel more detached and less inclined to make efforts to connect. In the same way, each person entering your life has their own hopes and expectations.

For example, a woman I know—let's call her Tyra—had one son. Tyra had always secretly desired a daughter. When her son married, she hoped that her son's partner would be the daughter she had always yearned to have. But Tyra's new daughter-in-law didn't feel the same way, for her life was absolutely filled with family, friends, and work. Tyra attempted to form a bonded relationship by sending small gifts, offering lunch dates, and sending occasional emails. Her daughter-in-law's responses were kind but aloof. Tyra ultimately acknowledged her disappointment and faced it with loving acceptance. This shift into self-awareness and acceptance allowed Tyra to embrace her daughter-in-law without overt or unconscious pressure. Through this graceful process, her daughter-in-law warmed to her over time.

Although Tyra's dream of having a daughter-in-law that felt like a true daughter may never materialize, her genuine acceptance of the situation has given Tyra freedom from angst. In this way, you can also come to notice and honor your hopes and needs. Simply allow yourself to acknowledge your desires and preferences, and then strive to relax with calm awareness. It is from a place of loving, powerful awareness that you will build greater respect for your own needs and the needs of others.

As you get to know the personalities of your "new" family in the years ahead, you may find that this relaxed, aware stance allows you to form healthier relationships that respect your needs and the needs of others. Over time, the relationships will blossom and mature based on the foundation of your wise, respectful awareness.

Wisdom Tip 47: Respect Your Adult Child's Parenting Style.

As your adult child learns to parent, allow the process to unfold. If you are asked for advice, feel free to chime in with your honest, respectful opinion. Otherwise, allow your adult child to parent in the ways that seem appropriate for them. The only exception, of course, would be times that you fear a parent's actions may ultimately put a child in emotional, mental, or physical danger. In such cases, it's important to have a direct, respectful conversation with your adult child in the most immediate way possible. (As always, any threat to a child's well-being should certainly be reported to authorities. Sadly, grandparents are often put into the position of protecting grandchildren or other children who cannot protect themselves.) In many cases, however, clashes result when grandparents comment on mostly harmless, if irritating and disrespectful, parenting behaviors.

One couple came to me after a family holiday dinner ended with their son and daughter-in-law leaving angrily with both children in tow. The wife had, with the best of intentions, simply asked that the toddler not be permitted to paint the walls with cranberry sauce. Their normally calm, thoughtful daughter-in-law became angry, accusing her mother-in-law of being judgmental and controlling. The holiday festivities unraveled from that point with threats that the young couple and their children would never return. Of course, it was appropriate for the grandmother to set reasonable boundaries regarding the cranberry sauce painting, but it seemed as if a bigger issue was at work.

During our session, my clients realized that they had been unconsciously criticizing their daughter-in-law's overall parenting style during their visits. The wife admitted to making her disapproval known in various ways, from edgy comments to gifts of parenting books. The husband also admitted to making occasional pointed comments regarding "how much parenting standards have changed." In retrospect, they saw that the cranberry sauce issue may have resulted from their daughter-in-law's pent-up response to feeling criticized.

The unpleasant experience offered a positive learning opportunity. It allowed the couple to see some of the judgmental, controlling behaviors they had unconsciously engaged in over time toward their son and daughter-in-law. This allowed the couple to give heartfelt apologies and move forward in healthier ways. In turn, the young couple apologized for their part in the holiday turmoil and the relationship ultimately improved on many levels. Clear boundaries, respect, and open communication were the keys.

Wisdom Tip 48: Be the Grandparent Your Grandchildren Need You to Be.

If you accept the role of grandparent with an open mind and heart, you may have the opportunity to share your love in the most beautiful way. Unfortunately, some come to the role of grandparenting with their own consious or unconscious agendas—such as wanting to control how their grandchildren are raised. If you want to enhance grandparenting to the fullest, the key is simple: put your own issues aside and be the grandparent that your grandchild needs you to be. By honoring the parents' rules and boundaries, you will give your grandchild the consistency that is needed.

Although occasional spoiling can be healthy if done in concert with the parents' approval, your grandchildren will feel confused if given mixed messages and inconsistent rules. As one of my friends confessed, "I wanted to shower my grandson with everything I didn't have to give my own kids. When my son left my grandson with me, I'd give in to his every whim. I loved doting on him—it was fun for me. But I realized after a few too many wake-up calls that my selfish behavior was harming my grandson, my son and his wife, and my relationships with all three."

In the end, your love, kindness, and consistency are your greatest gifts to your children and grandchildren.

Wisdom Tip 49: Learn to Let Go of Minor Issues.

As with other family issues, sometimes the best path is to release the issues that are simply unimportant. Many family issues arise from a battle of wills. When it comes down to it, most issues are not very critical in life. If one relative routinely shows up late to holiday events or another tends to forget to help in the kitchen, it can often be best to simply release any negativity around the situation. In most cases, adult children are rarely back at home for long. When they are home, set simple boundaries on the most important issues. For those issues that really aren't critical, allow yourself the gift of letting go.

One family was routinely miffed by an in-law's tendency to cancel on events at the last minute or simply be a "no show." Ultimately, they realized that they had no control over the situation and that it wasn't worth upsetting the evening. They chose to deal with the issue by setting a place at the table; if the inlaw arrived, they welcomed her. If she didn't arrive, they removed the place setting and let go.

As you look at the areas in your life negatively affected by family dynamics—and face them with wise awareness—you will find the power of graceful choice, acceptance, and release.

Embracing Changes within the Marital or Life Partner Relationship

It is often after children leave the nest or age begins to creep upward that the mid-life crisis rears its head. We often think of a mid-life crisis as being a blip around age forty-five or fifty that results in the purchase of a coveted sports car, a spending binge, or an adulterous affair. However, the stifled energy and emotions that result in a "mid-life" crisis can occur at any point in life—whether you are forty, sixty, or beyond. What is often perceived as a personal crisis is often actually a call from the soul for a reevaluation of life.

In our externally oriented society, we often assume that we can resolve pent-up unrest and angst by making an extravagant purchase, taking a whirlwind vacation, or seeking comfort in the arms of a different partner. On some level, it might be nice if it were that easy to effectively address such deep inner angst, yet the soul requires quite a lot more in the way of care and attention. If the soul's call is ignored or covered over with a fancy new car or sexual affair, the inner unrest remains and festers. Given the nature of relationships, it is in marriage and other intimate partnerships that the effects of mid-life transitions are often felt and displayed.

If you are in a life partnership, the period up to your sixties and beyond may bring you to seriously reevaluate your relationship with your partner. Whether you are married or in another love relationship, this era of your life can bring time for introspection and desired change. You and your partner may both be facing retirement; this may bring more time together—proximity and contact that may be desired or not. You might even come to a place where you feel a lack of love or affection for your partner—a sense that the relationship is no longer viable. You may be facing other adjustments with your partner, such as significant changes in health or age-related shifts in libido. Financial issues may come to the forefront as prices continue to rise and income-producing days fade. It is common for fear to well up surrounding the myriad life issues and worries that tend to arise. The tendency is to hide from the concerns—to push them aside and plug along. However, it is only through honest soul-searching that you can come to terms with the various changes taking place in your life.

After gaining greater awareness, you can begin heartfelt communication with your partner regarding your hopes, fears, and desires. When honesty and respect are honored, there is no ache or fear that cannot be openly addressed. Many partnership issues can be managed and even resolved through open communication and, when necessary, outside psychotherapeutic support. However, if you press down your fears and let yourself remain stuck and constrained, you will not be able to embrace and enjoy this next amazing era of your life. By addressing your fears and worries, you will be able to move forward with a free and open heart.

Given that divorce affects many women in their later years, this significant issue must be addressed openly. However, it's important to emphasize that marriage is a sacred contract and that divorce shouldn't be taken lightly or as a first-line solution. However, given the reality of divorce, it is necessary to pragmatically address this issue in a gentle, clear manner. The purpose of this section is not to advocate one life path over another. The purpose is to help you choose, with conscious awareness and wisdom, the path that is right and true for you. By acknowledging and accepting your decisions and the impact they will have, you may discover newfound clarity and ease. In this way, your conscious choices (whatever they may be) can guide you into making the most of the beautiful years ahead.

Wisdom Tip 50: Write a Heartfelt Letter to Your Partner.

Innermost thoughts and feelings can be difficult to ferret out, especially when fear and anxiety are at work. By writing a letter to your partner—a letter that is actually for your eyes only—you will be able to sort out some of your thoughts and feelings. *This letter is not intended to be read by or sent to your partner*; it is an exercise in private self-reflection.

In this process, allow yourself to write in a free-flowing way without censure or worry for grammar and sentence structure. Create a safe and relaxed place for your writing experience. Allow yourself to write about whatever comes to mind, be it joys, triumphs, regrets, resentments, fears, worries, or dreams for the future. After you've completed the letter, seal it and put it away for a few days. When you feel ready, re-read your letter. Let yourself notice the thoughts and emotions that arise. If you feel the need for further reflection and self-clarity—particularly if the contents of your letter press you toward significant life changes—you may wish to write a second letter to your partner. This one, too, is intended to allow you to contemplate and express your enduring, innermost thoughts and feelings. Again, seal the letter and read it a few days later.

This process will help you evaluate and clarify your relationship concerns and your hopes for the future of your relationship and its role in your life. The following are two brief, contrasting examples of letters written to partners:

First Example Letter to Partner

Dear Edward,

Time has flown by, hasn't it? I remember the first time I saw you in the cafe; I was so young, yet I felt in my heart that we would share a lifetime of love and devotion. Now, thirty-two years later, I feel like a fool. I have been a loving, devoted wife and mother. You have not been a loving, devoted husband and father. Although others see our marriage as a shiny, bright success, I know that it is dirty and tarnished by an endless series of broken promises and the dark resentments that have taken up residence.

With the children gone, the house seems dark and littered with loss. I've no distractions to keep me from the truth any longer. You have broken my heart one too many times. No. That's not accurate. You have broken my heart three thousand too many times. I have forgiven your ongoing emotional affair with work and your physical affairs with women, but the pain and resentment seem to linger and fester. Forgiveness does not wipe out my memories, my emotions, and the truth of who you are and what you have done to our life together.

Therapy has not helped us. It came too late and did too little. Now, when I see you, I see only lies and false dreams. I need and want to set myself free. One part of me tells me it's too late to start over, but that voice has been saying that for too many years. I know my life will change drastically and that our children and friendships will be affected, but I want a life that feels clean and true. I want and need a life without you in it. That's my truth.

Just writing these words makes my heart feel lighter and free. I want to say that I am sorry, but I'm not. I want to say that I'm crying as I write these lines, but I'm not. I feel as if a fresh breeze is sweeping through me. I know that this is right for me. It will be hard to start fresh so late in life, but it is the right path for me.

Sincerely,

Vanessa

Second Example Letter to Partner

Dear Nicholas,

Life gets so busy, and this pause helps me realize how rarely I make the time to reflect on what is most important to me. Today, I am making space to write to you, my dear life companion.

I want to thank you for being my lover and best friend. You have seen me and our family through so much. You have been my partner in child-rearing, creating a home filled with love, and so many life challenges. It was your unwavering love and support that saw me through the hardships of breast cancer. It was your love and conviction that pulled me through my life-changing auto accident. It was your unfaltering love that helped our family thrive through our son's drug addiction and recovery. It was your loving wisdom and can-do attitude that allowed us to handle a multitude of other parenting challenges as a cohesive team. With your kind heart and ever-present smile, you've seen our family through financial challenges, health problems, growing pains, and losses of faith.

Whether helping me return to college or supporting my work endeavors, you've always been in my corner. It's incredible to me that you somehow always managed to be in three places at once—at my side, behind me, and in front of me. You have been my friend, supporter, and guide when needed. Here I sit, on the cusp of turning sixty-two, and I know my life has been terrifically blessed by your presence. Where others might fear getting older, the prospect of getting older with you fills me with more joy than trepidation. Why? Because your love is unconditional. You see my beauty despite my crow's feet, age spots, and loosening skin. You touch my scars as if they are sweet rose petals.

Even as I write, I can hear your gentle voice as you run your fingers through my graying hair and say, "My sweetheart, gray hair looks marvelous on you." I can feel your fingers on my skin as you rub me at night and whisper, "Ah, the soft curves of your body get sexier every day." Possibly my favorite moments are those when you look into my eyes and say, "Our life together has been incredible, but growing older with you—having you all to myself—gets better every day."

I don't tell you enough how much these little things mean to me—maybe because they are not so little; they are bigger than my heart can properly express in words. So, darling, maybe my goal for our next few decades is to share with you—and with others—some of the extraordinary gifts you've given to me.

Love,

Kate

Wisdom Tip 51: Write a Heartfelt Letter to Yourself.

After you have completed your letter-writing process to your partner, give yourself the gift of writing a letter to yourself. To give your heart and mind the opportunity to digest and integrate the contents of your letter to your partner, you may wish to wait a day or more before taking this next step.

When you are ready to proceed, create a safe and relaxed space for your writing time. Allow this letter to be a nonjudgmental outpouring of your thoughts and feelings regarding your relationship with your partner, as well as other aspects of your inner world that may arise. Your letter may even hint at a vision of your future.

This process may prove to be very healing and empowering, for it will build on the substance and energy of the letter written to your partner. Indeed, it is through these very intimate personal processes that you can allow your psyche to flush out aspects that may have been repressed or overlooked. After your writing is complete, seal the letter and read it in a few days' time. If you feel drawn to write a second letter to yourself, repeat the same process.

It takes great courage to engage in this journey, so remember to be kind and gentle with yourself during this process.

As you notice the fruits of your work, you will begin to feel lighter and freer. You may not have any specific answers or directions, but you are well on your way. As a follow-up to the letters to your partner, the following are examples of letters written to the self:

First Example Letter to Self

Dear Vanessa,

I am questioning myself hourly. I know the path ahead— the path to leaving my marriage—will not be easy. I am a fixture in Edward's life, and he won't want to let me go. Yet each time I question myself, I re-read my letter to him. That letter reminds me of my truth. It gives me courage. When my scared voice comes up to taunt me about financial issues, fears of losing friends, or the tremendous energy it will take to set up a new household, I pull out my letter to Edward. It reminds me of my choices. I can stay and live in a house of resentment and anger. I can remain married to a man who never really sees me. I am familiar with this sad life. I also have the option to move forward and create a new life for myself, one that will give me space to discover who I am. This is a scary, unfamiliar path, but it calls to me constantly.

From this perspective, my choice is clear. I must move forward. I believe the kids will understand. My true friends won't turn their backs on me. My brother and sisters will surely support me. I know that this is right for me. I feel it in my bones. Most importantly, I feel it in my heart. I feel claustrophobic and contaminated in my marriage, and it is time to set myself free. No matter what lies ahead, it will be better than where I am now. I have the power and the courage to move forward. I want to spend the next years of my life finding myself and living for myself. A strong, gentle voice is whispering to me, "Everything will be okay."

I am crying now. Tears are slipping down my cheeks. They are tears of fear. They are tears of courage. They are tears of release.

Love,

Vanessa

Second Example Letter to Self

Dear Kate,

My heart is filled with gratitude. Life has surely brought its share of challenges my way, yet I have had countless more blessings than trials. When I think of the years that have disappeared behind me, I have no regrets. I have learned so much and have loved so deeply.

I have also been loved beyond my wildest imaginings. The love I have known from Nicholas has filled my days for the past thirty-seven years. His rare brand of love has been my oxygen and sunshine. I have never had to doubt the depth of his fidelity or love.

My children, family, and friends have also showered me with love. I sometimes ask myself, "Who are you, Kate, to have been so blessed by such rich love?" I know how fortunate I am. When I look at my life with all its blessings and learnings, I have no desire to relive my past or chase some vision of youth. Truly, I am grateful to be peering into my later years, for I have much more to discover and experience in days that wait in front of me.

Something new is calling my name. Something that tells me that this next stage is my time to venture and grow wildly. These coming years will give me the time, energy, and focus to give back just a fraction of the goodness that life has given to me. I can envision wrapping Nicholas in the folds of ever sweeter love. I can see our partnership growing more delightful as we cross little items off our bucket list. I can imagine my dormant adventurous side coming out as Nicholas and I explore life together. I want to accept Nicholas's invitation to join him in volunteering at the homeless shelter. I envision sewing, gardening, and baking to my heart's content. I imagine sitting on the porch at day's end with Nicholas at my side. All of this, and so much more, waits for me.

    Love,
    Kate

Wisdom Tip 52: Make a List of Your Relationship Goals.

As a result of writing your letters, you may have become more in tune with changes you would like to make. You may now be ready to formulate an outline of the specific changes and goals you envision. Be as specific as possible when you create your list. The more concrete and detailed your list, the more likely you are to take the necessary steps to follow through with your desires.

For example, your list might include a specific timeline for certain goals, a detailed list of items to discuss with your partner, and an outline of your relationship bucket list.

Wisdom Tip 53: Communicate Intentionally with Your Partner.

When you feel ready to discuss all that you have discovered, talk with your partner honestly, kindly, and respectfully. Of course, it's important to set a time to talk that is convenient and safe for both you and your partner. Know the purpose of your talk and your desired goals. Whether difficult or delightful in nature, it's important to speak your truth with courage and compassion. Allow your partner the opportunity to express personal thoughts and feelings.

When possible, make a vow to each other to work through issues as loving partners, and *always* with honesty, kindness, and respect. When faced with a challenging situation, remember that you cannot control your partner's behaviors; what you can control is your attitude, your conduct, and your personal boundaries.

Wisdom Tip 54: Meet with Your Primary Care Provider, Lawyer, and Financial Consultant to Address Important Issues.

Your sixties give you the perfect opportunity to fine-tune pragmatic issues with your partner. Many important concerns are avoided out of fear or resistance. Yet health issues, and even death, can strike at any age. This is the time to schedule intensive medical check-ups for you and your partner. If you have avoided it in the past, now is the time to make certain that you have appropriately addressed legal issues, such as wills, trusts, and medical directives like the Advance Healthcare Directive, Medical Power of Attorney, DNR (do not resuscitate) order, POLST (Physician Orders for Life-Sustaining Treatment), and organ donor forms. It can be frightening to address these issues, for they signify human mortality, yet to avoid tending to such issues can result in tremendous, unintentional harm to yourself and loved ones.

In the same way, financial issues are best faced head-on. Whether you have plenty of money or barely enough to cover your bills, it's important not to put your head in the sand. The money you invest in a consultation with a reputable financial advisor can do wonders in helping you feel safe and secure.

Wisdom Tip 55: Embrace Outside Support to Gain Clarity.

If you are struggling with new or historical partnership issues, this may be the perfect time to gain perspective by seeking outside support. Sometimes relationships simply get stagnant or hit low points that can be readily addressed within the partnership. In other cases, professional guidance is necessary to obtain objective insights. Whether you choose to seek guidance from a psychotherapist, support group, clergy member, spiritual advisor, or trusted mentor, remember that resources are available. Indeed, women's groups are often excellent forums for gaining support; you may find great wisdom and reassurance by listening and sharing with women who often have very similar life experiences.

It is important that you pay attention to any tendencies to self-isolate or anesthetize your fears by using substances or other forms of avoidance. Contemplating change can be difficult and scary, yet it might be exactly what you really want and need. As you evaluate your partnership and other life issues, it's important to have outside support. You deserve to gain the insights and clarity you need to move forward joyfully.

Wisdom Tip 56: Move Forward in Love.

Whatever choices you find before you and whatever decisions you make, do your utmost to come from a place of love. Envision this as a time to "clean house" and freshen up your world. By embracing a positive attitude, you can set the stage for a joy-filled future. Strive, in whatever choices you make, to act from a place of courage, dignity, and respect for yourself and others. In this way, you will create the life changes that you want with the utmost love and grace.

The Pain and Wisdom of Ending a Dead Relationship

It's the most natural thing in the world to want a relationship to last forever; on a visceral level, we often hope to remain in a loving, connected, and committed relationship for a lifetime. Sadly, this is not always the case for partnerships. For a wide variety of reasons (some of which you may have explored in your letter-writing earlier) one or both partners may find the need or desire to end a relationship.

Such endings are not to be taken lightly, for incredible pain and grief can come with such partings. Of course, there are times that the most difficult part of ending a relationship is knowing when the relationship is dead and when it still has hope. It is important to spend the necessary time and energy to explore this aspect before making a big life decision. One of the reasons for doing this is to avoid taking old, unresolved relationship baggage into your new life. Another valid reason is to ensure that you know you have done all that you can to make things right in light of your commitments. It's also tremendously important to ensure that you've done the necessary soul-searching to know what you need and want in the next phase of your life; otherwise, you risk leaving a relationship only to stagnate in old thoughts and patterns.

There are certainly situations where partners have invested in diligent soul-searching and have done everything possible to enliven the relationship, only to find themselves at a stalemate. In these cases, ending the relationship may be the wisest choice of all. Of course, there are times when one partner is finished with the relationship and the other is not. Even in cases where agreement is minimal and emotions run high, the situation can be handled with respectful grace. As well, no matter how friendly the parting may be, the process can be quite painful and emotional. Trust, as you move forward, that the pain will subside and allow room for new growth and joyful delights.

Wisdom Tip 57: Know Your Wants, Needs, and Key Goals as You Move Forward.

If you elect to end your current partnership, it's important to be honest with yourself about your list of "wants." Your list may include how you want the relationship to conclude; some individuals prefer an abrupt shift, whereas others prefer to move slowly. It's also vital that you know what type of relationship you envision for you and your soon-to-be former partner. Do you want a close friendship, occasional contact, or do you prefer no contact at all?

In addition, it's vital that you know your desires in regard to pragmatic issues, such as housing, furnishings, insurance, automobiles, property, savings, and retirement accounts. Once you have clarified your list of wants, you will then be in a position to share the information openly and honestly with your partner.

This same procedure applies to your needs. It's important that you know what you *need* in order to move into this next phase of your life. You may need financial support. You may need to create a list of all material items built up during the relationship. If poor boundaries have been an issue, you may need to create strong boundaries. You may need to find a safe place to stay (or ask your partner to leave) if you are not feeling safe and respected. A clear list of your needs will help you move forward with greater assurance.

In the same way, a clear list of goals will be very helpful during the transition. A clear, but somewhat flexible, timeline will help you move forward steadily and surely. For example, if finding a new home is a key goal, it would be helpful to have sub-goals, such as investigating the areas you prefer, determining a suitable home price and style, and finding the right real estate agent. As a part of each sub-goal is accomplished, you will feel that much closer to achieving one of your key goals and creating the new life you desire. If you need a boost, revisit "Nine Steps for Empowered Change" in Chapter 2.

Wisdom Tip 58: Make "Honesty, Patience, and Loving Kindness" Your Mantra.

Divorce and other relationship endings can bring out the worst in partners. When both parties are angry, resentful, and bitter, the results can be extremely costly and emotionally damaging. In cases where only one partner is filled with hostility, the results can also be disastrous. As a result, the wisest course is to strive to be free of negativity. Even if your soon-to-be former partner is angry and hostile, strive not to engage. In doing so, you will not only avoid fueling your partner's rage, you will also save yourself the heart-ache and toxicity of being drawn into the fray.

Of course, this does not mean that you cave in to your partner's demands or let someone take advantage of you. It simply means that you know your wants, needs, and goals and strive to achieve them with honesty, patience, and loving kindness. It also means that you stick firmly to what is most important to you and work to be flexible on the less important matters.

Wisdom Tip 59: Seek the Support of True Friends and Step Back from Non-Friends.

Friendships are often tested most when couples part ways. There are friends who overtly choose one partner, whereas others strive to take a middle ground. Some friends step away out of fear of "taking sides." Indeed, it is not uncommon for some married friends to discontinue contact altogether out of fear of "catching" the divorce virus or getting involved in some way. Whatever the dynamics may be, strive to face them with awareness and acceptance.

Life has a way of separating the wheat from the chaff during the most challenging times. In this way, you will have the gift of discovering which friendships are true and stalwart and which friendships may not have been friendships at all. It will be in the embrace and wise counsel of your true friends that you will find the strength, courage, and support necessary to build the new life you are seeking.

Wisdom Tip 60: Invest in Psychotherapy to Obtain Healing Guidance and Support as You Journey Forward

Psychotherapy can be incredibly helpful both during and after the ending of a relationship. A skilled psychotherapist can offer objective, insightful support, while also helping you work through unresolved personal issues.

If finances or other issues prevent you from seeking individual psychotherapy, options such as group therapy, religious support, and appropriate online forums can be beneficial. Group therapy can be particularly helpful during relationship transitions, for group members often feel validated when sharing and listening to perspectives of those in similar situations.

The support and self-awareness you gain as a result of your efforts will be well worth any money, time, and effort expended.

Wisdom Tip 61: Strive for Mediation when Possible.

Relationship dissolutions often involve significant assets. When stubbornness and hot tempers come into play, reason often goes out the window. In such cases, the tendency is to run directly to an attorney who will outwit and outperform the opposing counsel. Sadly, this attitude reduces the couple's assets as it builds the attorneys' bank account. The wisest of partners put their egos aside and work together to move forward without costly attorney and legal fees. An excellent mediator can save you time, money, and an exhausting legal battle. Of course, both partners must want to engage in meditation for it to be effective. When possible, work with your partner to mediate—rather than litigate—your dissolution.

Wisdom Tip 62: Hold Fast to Moving Forward with Integrity.

As you move into your new life, do so with positive intentions and positive behaviors. Although periods of transition can be intensely challenging and negatively trigger even the kindest, most even-tempered souls, it is important to stay true to your better self. When you make choices that align with your moral code and beliefs, you will be able to be pleased with yourself in the long term. You will build true self-esteem as you put your energy into creating positive, empowering thoughts and behaviors.

Although the outcome may not always be what is truly fair or what you would hope for, your integrity is priceless. As long as you hold onto your integrity, you will know that you have come out exactly where you need to be; a woman who is true to herself—true to her integrity.

Dating Joyfully

Many women choose to stay single in their more mature years. This is a wonderful, and often freeing, option for an increasing number of women. Rather than seeking a lifelong partner or utilizing energy to date, some women channel their full energy into their own lives. When this choice is made from a place of peace and openness, it can lead to incredible years filled with personal pursuits, self-growth, and vast joy. The key, of course, is to make certain that your choices (whatever they may be) are made in a non-reactive way that stems from clarity and self-love. The best choices are made with a clean, healed heart, for choices made from a place of fear often limit a woman's personal fulfillment. Whether you choose to date or not is your choice, and one that deserves your wise attention.

If you choose to engage in dating after a long-term relationship ends, it is often very helpful to refrain from dating for at least one year. This period allows for soul searching, healing, and renewal. Sacred spaces after major life transitions provide the opportunity to thoughtfully reflect, learn valuable lessons from the experience, and recalibrate. If this period is spent in distracted behavior, anger, or resentment, true healing will not be possible. Of course, bouts of sadness and anger are a natural part of grieving, so it is important to honor the feelings that arise; it is equally important to process the feelings and let them move outward. If the feelings get "stuck" inside of you, your healing process will stagnate. It is for this reason that some people do not heal even many years after a relationship has ended; if the years are spent in negativity or avoidant behaviors (e.g., speed dating, self-isolation, substance use, etc.), then the healing process simply does not occur no matter how much time has passed.

In addition, older women often note that they feel extremely defensive and fearful of the dating process. This can be a natural response after experiencing significant hurts, sorrows, and betrayals throughout many decades. The fears that arise, which are often unconsciously built up over time, often result in the unconscious formation of fear-based defenses to avoid emotional connection. As protective as these types of defensive armor may feel, they often lead to behaviors that silently (or not-so-silently) push others away. A defense may feel helpful, yet it is a double-edged sword. Defenses can keep others at bay *and* lock a woman inside herself. An unhealed heart (and the internal immobilization that results) can be reflected in attitudes and behaviors that are often generally unhelpful in the dating world.

And so, if you desire to first work on healing yourself in whatever arenas speak to you—women's groups, individual therapy, bibliotherapy, somatic work, or otherwise— it will allow you to understand yourself, detox, and build your own sense of power. As a result, your vital sense of self-esteem will feel strong and expansive. You will know when you are ready to date again, for you will feel a peaceful sense of confidence and graceful ease. This sense of readiness may be tinged with an edge of anxiety, but that is only natural.

No matter your age, today's dating world can be a scary place. Even for those who are young, it seems increasingly difficult to meet a potential partner in an organic way. Whether striving to connect with others in the online realm, through social activities, or by chance, the mere thought of "starting again" can be intimidating. When it comes to dating in one's later years, a host of age-related fears often make the idea of dating even more anxiety-inducing. Many women share their dating fears with me, and all of their fears are understandable, normal, and very real to them. By sharing some of their stories, you may realize that your fears are not unique and that you are not alone.

Let's look at Lilli, age sixty-seven, who found herself in the dating world after forty-one years of marriage. In red-cheeked embarrassment, Lilli confessed, "I am so afraid. I want to date and find a partner to share this next part of my life with, but I'm terrified. My husband is the only man who has seen me naked for over forty years. I was thin and sexy when I met him. We grew flabby and wrinkly together; it was normal and no big deal. My breasts feel like they droop down to my knees, my skin is as wrinkled as an elephant's, and my waistline is double what it was forty years ago. I can't imagine taking my clothes off in front of some other man. He'd probably scream and run away before we even got to sex. And that's another problem altogether; my sex drive is all but gone."

My honest response reassured her. "I hear how scared you are, Lilli," I said. "It may help to know that many women I work with express similar fears. It's very natural to be afraid of something so unfamiliar and new."

After we talked for a bit, I asked her if she'd like to hear a humorous thought on the matter. With an anxious smile, she nodded her head. I told her this truth:

"I work with men also, and they tell me their fears as well. Older men have their own set of anxieties. They feel flabby, wrinkled, and old. They worry about their libido, ability to get erections, and how their breasts and testicles sag. The similarities are endearing and humorous—older men are scared too."

"Really?" Lilli questioned with a halfsmile.

"Yes, Lilli," I responded, "Men also have their fears and worries."

Another poignant tale offers insight in another common dating fear. With her divorce two years behind her, Belinda, age sixty-five, decided that she was ready to date again. Belinda was terrified of entering the dating world for many reasons, including the fact that she has genital herpes, a common sexually transmitted disease (STD). Although she was often asymptomatic, Belinda was terrified that a "good man" would reject her as a result of her STD, yet she didn't want to hide the truth from a potential partner.

Belinda found the courage to begin dating and was honest about her situation with the men she dated. A few were scared off, and their apparent rejections hurt Belinda quite deeply. But Belinda continued to date, and she ultimately met a few men who accepted her situation without much concern. Now with a gentleman whose company, friendship, and sexuality she enjoys, Belinda says, "It was worth the wait!"

JoJo, age sixty-one, offers a dramatic example of another fairly common issue. Married three times, JoJo began toying with the idea of dating while her divorce was being finalized. She felt that she was ready to move forward with an open, positive attitude. However, after anxiously completing an online profile on a popular dating site with her daughter's help, JoJo found herself avoiding her computer. Confused and angry, JoJo came to see me.

"I don't know what's wrong with me," she said. "All of a sudden I'm furious about the whole dating thing. I hate men. I don't want to date. Every man I have been with has taken advantage of me, lied, or cheated on me. I don't know why I feel compelled to date again. I feel like I have to have a man to be complete—to share my life with—but I can't bear the thought of actually being with one of them. The thought of kissing a man makes my skin crawl."

Clearly, JoJo was not at all ready to venture into the dating world. As she discovered, it was far better to turn her attention inside herself to heal the source of her deep anger and resentment. Through individual therapy and group work, JoJo is slowly moving forward; however, the significant emotional scars from her negative relationship experiences will take time and focused energy to heal.

It can be difficult to move forward after the ending of any relationship, yet the sorrow can feel heavier and more solitary when a woman is in her later years. Age has a way of making a woman feel more isolated, for many friends are married (happily or otherwise) and engaged in lives of their own. Yet there are many women in the same position—women who have left their relationships or whose partners have passed away. It is in the company of these other single women that you can often find support and friendship as you heal and re-envision your future.

Wisdom Tip 63: Take Your Time Deciding When and If to Date.

You might initially feel that you never want to date or be in a romantic relationship again. You may ultimately change your mind, or you may elect to remain single. Although you might feel pressure from yourself, family, or friends to date again, remember that it is both okay and necessary to take your time.

Wisdom Tip 64: Explore Various Opportunities When Seeking a Romantic Partner.

Remember that there are many ways to meet potential partners. Whether you take dancing classes, join a hiking club, attend religious gatherings, or frequent cultural events, follow your heart in embracing the greater world. As you meet new people at these venues, you will begin forming new friendships based on shared interests.

Wisdom Tip 65: Move with Awareness into the World of Online Dating.

If you choose to date online, proceed slowly. Complete any online questionnaire honestly, offering current photos and accurate infor-mation. If you elect to meet someone in person, let a friend know the meeting place, time, and personal details. I always suggest to clients that the first few meetings be time-limited (a half hour or so) and take place in a coffee shop or other public setting.

Wisdom Tip 66: Attend to Your Instincts and Red Flags as You Date.

As you are getting to know someone, listen to your gut. Notice any "red flags," such as the person chronically arriving late for meetings, being self-absorbed, or engaging in generally rude behavior. If a person is unkind or disrespectful during the dating process, the situation will likely worsen over time. You deserve to be treated with respect!

Wisdom Tip 67: Honor Yourself—NEVER Apologize or Make Excuses for Who You Are.

Resist any inclination to apologize for not looking different (e.g., thinner, more fit, or younger) than you do. Do your best to present yourself in a way that feels right to you. Whatever your personal preference and style (clothes, hair, and any makeup), let yourself be who you are. Let your attitude reflect that you are comfortable and proud of every inch and fiber of your being. Never apologize or make excuses for being your beautiful, mature self.

Wisdom Tip 68: Know and Respect Your Personal Boundaries.

You might be tempted to act in certain ways or accept certain behaviors out of fear of being rejected or being left single. Clear boundaries delineate an individual's needs and preferences regarding respectful, appropriate behavior (e.g., sexuality, personal space, personal information, finances, etc.). It's important to know what your boundaries are and then stick to them. When you come from a place of self-respect and clear boundaries, you are more likely to find a suitable, respectful partner.

Wisdom Tip 69: Laugh, Laugh, Laugh at the Wild Ways of Life.

Don't take dating too seriously. Find the humor in the wild world of partner searching. If you are anxious or nervous, remember that your date is likely feeling much the same way. When in doubt, make a gentle joke about your unease.

As one newly sixty-two-year-old client noted, "When I told my dinner date that it just didn't seem right to be dating as a senior citizen, he laughed and said, 'I understand completely. Imagine how I feel at seventy-two! It's just crazy; my father was at home in a rocking chair at my age.'" The awkwardness evaporated and that evening began the start of a lovely, later-life romance.

Wisdom Tip 70: Seek Support as You Navigate the World of Dating.

The topic of dating is often a hot issue in my weekly women's support group. This confidential forum provides the opportunity to share and connect with other women who are experiencing similar issues. It's common for the women to venture into the dating world and then bring their experiences back to the group for a "reality check." Many clients have noted that group therapy provides the perfect opportunity to be validated and obtain guidance by listening to the shared issues and common themes that arise.

Whether you talk with friends, create a coffee group, attend individual psychotherapy, or seek group therapy, remember to seek support as you explore the dating world.

Wisdom Tip 71: Embrace the Idea that You Don't NEED a Partner to Find Joy.

As you heal from past hurts, you will find great love for yourself. You will find that you are worthy, beautiful, and loveable. You will also find that you don't need a mate to "complete" you. You may elect to choose a mate to share your life with, but you will find that this is just one possible option. As you age joyfully, you will find that a healthy, radiant YOU is "the one" who completes you.

Let yourself move into this next era of your life with true freedom. Let yourself know that, although you are valuable at any age, you have more to offer now than ever. You have wisdom, courage, and grace. Every wrinkle and laugh line is a testament to the tremendous life you have lived and the wisdom you have earned. Know this truth, and wear it with a proud, welcoming smile.

CHAPTER 6

A Brave, Passionate You

The Light Within: You and Your Internal Power

As we bring our journey together into another phase, let me remind you of your internal power. It's your greatest asset; it is the light—the energy—of who you are. Every woman's internal power is hers alone to understand, explore, and nourish.

I envision my own internal power as a force that is constantly being refined, enlivened, and strengthened. The source of my internal power is a blend of passion, love, integrity, internal wisdom, humility, divine essence, courage, resilience, determination, perseverance, and good will. These qualities (and many more) are the fuel that allow my inner light to radiate with strength. There are times when my internal power feels strong and deep, and there are other times when it feels a bit fragile. I have come to know that this is not a weakness within me; it is the natural course of life. Those moments and periods of fragility are, indeed, the times the divine seems to say, "You are ready for yet another test. You are ready to take another step forward—another step upward—in your journey. You've the courage, resilience, and power to make it through. Access your inner resources. Reach out to your external resources. Connect with your higher power. You will come out the other side stronger and wiser than ever before. Have faith that all will be well."

Let me share a secret with you: Whereas the aging process might lead us to experience many losses in life, internal power is not one of them. A key benefit of aging is that one's internal power can grow wildly with each passing year. When you face life with an attitude of intentionality and conscious awareness, when you honor and nourish your internal power, it increases in strength and magnitude. This may certainly be one of the most profound blessings in life.

What is your internal power? It's important for you to know what "internal power" means to you, for this is the inner source that feeds you. Your internal power may have been marginalized, ignored, or misunderstood for much of your life. Now is your time to explore it, breathe into it, and allow it to bring your entire being into greater focus. All of the work you have done in the earlier chapters will allow you to better understand and foster this most precious power.

Wisdom Tip 72: Explore Your Vision of Internal Power.

Write out a personalized definition of what internal power means to you. Factors such as your personality, life experiences, attitudes, and beliefs converge to create a sense of internal power that is unlike any other's. In writing your own definition, you will come to better understand the nature of your inimitable internal power. You may find yourself rewriting and fine-tuning your definition; take as long as you like to create and recreate a description that feels right to you.

Wisdom Tip 73: Feel the Strength of Your Internal Power.

Now that you have a description of your internal power, it's time to truly feel that internal power within your own being. Imagine a time that you felt powerful; envision a situation that gave you the opportunity to feel truly strong from within. If you like, close your eyes and again imagine that situation. Notice where in your body you felt that power. Did your strength emanate from your solar plexus? Your heart? Your stomach? The crown of your head? Or is it somewhere else in your body? Perhaps you sensed it in several areas at once?

Observe the feelings and the place in your body where you felt a sense of power. This area (or areas) may be the center of your internal power. When you are aware of where you *feel* your internal power, you will be able to better access that power in times of intensity, crisis, or unrest.

When I began my journey into the life of my dreams, I was often uncertain. I found myself unsteady at times, much like a newborn colt who is struggling for strength and stability. I continued forward, building my inner strength by trial and error. A pivotal moment came as the result of giving yet another presentation before my doctoral colleagues. Although I had initially been shaky and anxious about speaking to these formidable groups, I no longer had butterflies in my stomach before, during, and after various mandatory presentations. Following a particularly complex presentation, a fellow student offered her congratulations. Her kind words were appreciated, yet it was her last comment (a seeming afterthought) that was unforgettable.

She noted, "I've watched you grow so much over the years. During your presentation, I noticed that you kept touching your solar plexus, particularly when you were passionate about an issue. It's a gesture that I've never seen you make before."

I was grateful and intrigued by her insight, for I soon learned that this was my power center—my touchstone space for affirming and accessing my inner strength. By unconsciously touching my power center, I was talking to and accessing my internal power, and it was talking reassuringly back to me.

Your internal power is accessible to you. At first, all you need do is become aware of it and attuned to it. With care and attention, you will be able to nourish and strengthen your internal power. Like a physical muscle, the more you attend to it—the more you access it and utilize it—the stronger and more powerful it will become. Remember, this internal power isn't available to just certain people; it is within every person. It is already within you, waiting to be honed and strengthened at every opportunity.

Wisdom Tip 74: Cultivate Greater Internal Power with Awareness.

You can nurture your internal power by tuning in to yourself. When you are feeling powerful, observe the situation. Notice how and where you feel powerful in your body during such times. Note the thoughts, attitudes, and behaviors that are feeding this sense of power. Strive to bring the same powerful energy to other situations and areas of your life.

You can also nurture your internal power by noticing when you feel powerless or fragile. Notice how and where in your body you feel fragile or weak. Observe the thoughts, attitudes, and behaviors that are feeding the sense of powerlessness or fragility. Then pause to breathe. Pause to access your internal power. Pause to shift your thoughts, attitudes, and behaviors to create a more powerful you. Pause in gratitude for your internal power. The more you notice, nourish, and access it, the stronger it will grow.

One final note about your internal power: internal power is *not* the same thing as aggression or force. In fact, true internal power comes from a place of inner peace and strength. Internal power is respectful, dignified, focused, and firm. Of course, it has the capacity to uplevel to fierceness when necessary, yet it is not aggressive or domineering in nature. Internal power can, at times, be confused with destructive forms of power, yet constant awareness and practice will help you differentiate.

Make Poetry: You and Your Passion

Your journey through this book has, I pray, given you greater awareness of your own gorgeous, powerful inner light. It is my hope that you've also become more attuned to what gives you joy. Indeed, life's challenges may have left you not knowing joy or feeling as though you "lost" your sense of joy. Yet remember that joy is an eternal, internal flame that is sometimes bright and at other times barely flickering. Once we get to know what gives us joy—once we know what true joy feels like—we then have a sense of life as it is meant to be. From this space, we can create greater joy each day.

It is important to note that joy is far different from the fleeting, external happiness that is found in pleasure-seeking activities, such as accruing material wealth, buying endlessly, having meaningless sex, using drugs, drinking, etc. All of this is an endless, futile search for something outside the self. It's a precarious place to live, for if you rely on an external item or achievement to give you happiness, your happiness fades as soon as the "high" from that item or accomplishment has faded away.

A poignant story reflects the intersection of joy and personal power—of using these forces to find one's passions in life. The story that I bring to you is one of transformation from sadness and powerlessness to the beginnings of light, the growth of joy, and the precious knowing of passion. So let me introduce you to Naomi, a kind and gentle woman in her late fifties. Naomi might be easy to spot in a crowd, for she is lovely in a warm and genuine way, yet Naomi might also blend into a crowd for the very same reason; she is not one to advertise her own precious qualities. This is how Naomi has lived her entire life. She has been quiet, demure, and waiting in the background. Naomi has lived in a muted way that dulled her inner and outer being. It was Naomi's increasing sense of depression—triggered by looking ahead into the next phase of her life—that brought her to me.

As Naomi said, "I've always been on the quiet, reticent side. I don't like being the focus of attention. Even though I know I'm a good person, have made a good living, and have had a good, if not passionate, partner in my life, I realize now that my life has been flat and rather gray in color. I figured it was normal for me to feel somewhat glum most of the time with some occasional upticks—moments of feeling okay. Other than the periods of feeling slightly better than gray, I think that I've lived my life without real expression. I don't know a better way to phrase it, but I don't really know what it means to be joyful or happy. I want to know these feelings. I don't want to live feeling drab and gray for the rest of my life. I worry that if I don't address this now, the depression that's sneaking in will take me over. I don't want to be a sad, purposeless woman."

Naomi paused and our brown eyes met with deep understanding. She continued, "I don't know why I've had this epiphany. Maybe because I'm slowing down enough to notice. Maybe because I've lost a few close friends and am feeling the pain of that. Maybe it's because I want my life to matter. That's a big piece of it; I feel that my life doesn't matter, that my existence doesn't matter. If I disappeared off the face of the earth, only a few people would notice—my son, my partner, a few friends, and probably my boss. Other than that, I've not much to show for my life. That's a sad thing to say, but it's true."

Naomi looked at the ground and then back into my eyes. "I want to find some joy in my life. I want to know what joy feels like. I want my life to mean something to me. Can you help me?"

Over the course of many sessions, Naomi and I worked to discover what brought her joy. Having never known real joy, it was a hard task for Naomi to discover what might make her smile inside. Of course, she was highly competent in the job she'd held for nearly thirty years. Naomi gave devoted effort to her partner and to the raising of their now-grown child. Yet as Naomi came to discover, her life was marked by endless periods of "doing the right thing," not by exclamation points of doing what might bring her joy. At one point, I asked Naomi if she recalled being joyful as a child. Her only memory of what might be called joy was hiding under the covers with her dog. It was in those quiet moments shared with her Old English sheepdog that Naomi felt a sense of joy. This memory was a good place from which to start.

At the end of one session, I asked Naomi to tend to a bit of "homework." The homework was simple: to notice anything and everything that gave her a sense of joy—no matter how small. At our next appointment a few weeks later, Naomi reported that she'd found joy by going outside for walks. She normally exercised inside, yet something urged her to begin taking walks every morning. In the course of her walks, Naomi found that something else gave her joy.

With a soft smile on her face, Naomi laughed, "I've found that I love picking up trash as I walk. Our neighborhood is busy, and we get loads of litter on the street. I've always sighed and complained to myself about it, but I've never done anything to address the constant eyesore. So I put on a pair of disposable gloves, grabbed a bag, and cleaned up as I walked. I can't tell you how amazing it felt. Maybe not so much right in that moment, but afterward—staring at the bag of trash as I put it in the bin—I felt happy. I was pleased with myself. Then it got even better. It seemed like people weren't littering like before, as though my cleaning efforts made it pretty enough that they didn't want to spoil it. Is that possible?"

I laughed gently and nodded, "Yes, it's surely possible. You were apparently a role model for your neighbors. People are less likely to litter or desecrate an area that is clean and tidy. Just like with graffiti. Mess breeds more mess, and litter breeds more litter. You did so much good for yourself and for others. Impressive!"

Naomi smiled and said, "I didn't know you could find joy in such little things. But there I was, feeling joyful. And I did what you suggested; I really paid attention to that joy and every other little thing I did that felt joyful. It's amazing. There's joy to be found in the tiniest of things. I even rescued a tiny lizard in the road. Something that simple gave me joy. I need to keep at it, because I'm slowly feeling as if I matter—even if it's in small ways like picking up litter or rescuing lizards."

Before too long, Naomi was ready to investigate one of joy's cousins: passion. When I brought up the subject, Naomi's brown eyes lit up with fear.

"Passion?" she queried. "I'm not a passionate person; I'm a quiet person. No, passion's not for me. That's surely out of my comfort zone."

I smiled and explained, "Passion is an interesting creature, Naomi. It's tied to joy. Once you've touched upon true joy, passion may begin to creep in naturally. You needn't fear passion. I see passion as joy with fiery wings. It's that simple. When you discover your joy and then put that joy into action, you are giving life to something sacred. Passion is joy channeled into the world through you. When combined with your internal power, passion allows you to live with a sense of real purpose. Not that you can't have purpose without passion, of course. It's just that passion and internal power bring purpose—whatever it may be—to life in an intense, almost explosive way."

Naomi's dark eyes widened. "Okay, I get that in my head, but I don't know what you mean. If you don't mind, could you tell me something that you are passionate about?"

I laughed and said, "Of course. I am passionate in this very moment. I am passionate about my work as a psychologist. I am passionate about helping others. I am passionate about writing. I am passionate about nature, animals, music, yoga, and laughing. I am passionate about cleaning up litter at the beach and on my daily walks. I am passionate about relationships. I am passionate about being a good role model. I am intensely passionate about respect and integrity. Those are just a few of my passions, Naomi, but I think that's a good enough start. Now that you know a few of my passions, let's see if we can find a few things that might create a sense of passion in you."

Naomi nodded her head and giggled. "Okay, that makes it less scary. I thought maybe I was going to have to go skydiving, move to India, or paint like Picasso. But I get it; passion can be felt in little, everyday things—just like joy."

I smiled and said, "Yes, exactly. Your homework, as you might imagine, will be to notice what gives you even the tiniest hint of passion."

Naomi came to her next appointment with a soft glow actually emanating from within her. I smiled but didn't comment on what I noticed. As the session unfolded, it became clear that Naomi took her homework very seriously. She not only tracked her feelings of passion, but she also tracked—and acted on—a few items that she felt passionate about. In the four weeks since I'd seen her last, Naomi had taken her self-work into her own hands.

As Naomi explained, "I realized that I have passion when it comes to easing suffering. I have passion when it comes to tiny babies. I have passion for animals—for helping them and caring for them. Strangely, I haven't had a pet since I was little, so the lack of that connection didn't really cross my radar. I also have a passion for wanting to change things. I can't stand hearing about the homeless in our area. I am actually afraid of the homeless population, but I am passionate about changing that—in myself and in the world—so I took action. I've started volunteering with a homeless shelter. I've gone twice already. It's hard and unsettling, but it's right for me. I feel a fire inside me when I help there. I know I'm doing good.

"And, get this, I know I have much more to do. I've just begun. I can feel a fire that wants to grow and help create change. I feel this. This is passion. This is it. This is what I've been missing all my life. My job and my family have been about devotion and about doing what I felt I *should* do. This is different. This is a cause that makes me feel alive, as if my efforts really matter. I can't express it any better. I just want more of *this* feeling."

I smiled, and our eyes met with deep understanding. "Yes, Naomi, I imagine that you do want more of *this,* which is passion come to life. Your energy is quite different when you talk about your passions. How does it feel to feel passionate about something?"

She laughed. "It feels exceptional. My heart knows the difference. It's doesn't feel gray; it's technicolor. Such a difference. And I'm doing something else. I've applied to adopt a three-year-old dog from a shelter, and it's a half Old English sheepdog. His name is 'Maximus.' I'm very excited. So I'm feeling joy and passion. It's lovely. It really is."

I smiled at Naomi and noted, "You are radiant, Naomi. You are shining from the inside out."

With a nonchalant shrug of her shoulders and a shy smile, Naomi said, "Funny you say that. I can't see it, but I surely can feel it. Thanks for noticing."

A few sessions later, Naomi's glow hadn't dimmed; it had only grown stronger. As if she were making up for fifty-some years of dreariness, Naomi was coming to life in way reminiscent of time-lapse photography; she was unfurling before my eyes.

In her quiet, gentle way, Naomi shared, "A new thought keeps coming to me now. I can't shake it. I know it is early in my work with the homeless, but it's very energizing for me. I feel very passionate about it and very committed. Here's how I know that it's truly important: I was never excited to retire before, but I'm thinking about it constantly, even though it's a few years away. It can't come soon enough because I want to do more work with the homeless—much more—when I retire. I love the passion I have in my life now. I love feeling joy. I love feeling that the moments and little things in life matter. I love feeling as though I have a purpose that is important. It feels like my life is taking shape for the first time—a shape I want it to take."

Indeed, Naomi was definitely creating shape in her life. Like all processes, it wasn't overnight. Yet that was part of the beauty. There was no instant transformation, only a slow turning from gray to color. It was a beautiful sight to see—a woman who transformed a gray-filled world to one of kaleidoscope, jewel-toned energy.

So as you set yourself free to embrace and enjoy this next phase of your life, trust that your journey is a process. Trust that every little positive change you make truly matters. Know that every shift you create will make way for another delightful opening. Allow the cascade to unfold before you. And trust, deep in your soul, that you are meant to shine and radiate as only you—a most incomparable, joyful woman—can do. Your journey may unfurl in ways that are similar to Naomi's, or your path may be very different. It's not the direction of the path that is important, for what is compelling and inviting to one person may not be interesting to another. What is critical here is that you allow yourself to blossom. This time of your life is all about being your most radiant, fulfilled "you."

You may have noticed that this section began with the words "Make Poetry." This heading came to me one early dawn as I was thinking about the remarkable process of aging. When we are younger, we are told what we *must* do. We are admonished about what we *can't* do. We are directed to do what we *should* do. We are forced to conform to what we are *required* to be. We are channeled to conform, often at the expense of our inner selves and our very souls. The promising little poet, the messy baker, the coloring-out-of-the-lines artist, the off-key singer, the would-be carpenter, the fledgling mechanic, and the tiny seamstress—all those nascent bits of our younger selves that are so full of promise and life—are buried or sent scurrying away. In many cases, these beautiful acorns of potential are replaced by droll uniformity and must-dos.

So I entreat you: This is the time to awaken those lost pieces of yourself. This is the time to unearth that which has been waiting for you for far too long. This is the time to write the most beautiful story. This is the time to make poetry within every aspect of your precious, sweet being. This is the time to make poetry of your life.

Wisdom Tip 75: Discover Your Passions in Life.

What are your passions? Have they changed over the course of your life, or are they still the same? Perhaps you already know your passions and perhaps you don't. If you are already fully aware of your passions, take the time to revisit them with gratitude.

If you don't know your passions at all or you don't know them very well, this is your opportunity to play and explore. Now is your opportunity to create a list of all the passions you have in life. Be as wild and creative as you like. Your passions do not need to be confined to something you have done or are actively doing. Your passions can include your most vivid longings and dreams.

Wisdom Tip 76: Foster Awareness of Your "Must" Passions.

As you look at your list of your passions, notice which ones are dormant or unlived. Notice which you might revisit and breathe into with fresh life and power. Notice those that seem to call out to you as though you "must" attend to them. These are the passions that are asking for your care and attention. It is these passions that want to be part of your joyful journey into aging.

Wisdom Tip 77: Envision Your Passions Exploding into Life.

Now is your time to get excited. Imagine your passions coming to life. Imagine creating or recreating whatever is desired and necessary to ignite your passions. Perhaps it's just an attitude adjustment that's needed. Maybe it's time to think outside the box. Perhaps now is your time to leave behind a wilting passion to free up your energy for something new.

If the changes you envision feel unwieldy, revisit "Nine Steps for Empowered Change" in chapter 2.

Wisdom Tip 78: Share Your Passions with Delight.

There's nothing like sharing our passions with others. As we talk about our passions, our inner fire can get even stronger. By inviting and allowing others to share in our passions, whether as our supporters or as beneficiaries of our efforts, the internal flame gets stronger. As you include others in your passions, you ignite the passion in others. Reach wide. Be inclusive. Share your passions in every way possible.

Great Dreams, Big Challenges, and Giant Opportunities: It's All in the Weaving

Dreams and passions sometimes intersect. Our dreams often hold our inner wishes and imaginings. In truth, some of our dreams are meant to come to life, whereas other dreams seem quite content to sit on the shelf as sweet imaginings. It's important to know the difference between the two. A simple test may help you understand the difference: If a dream calls to you as a "must," as a thing that you must accomplish or experience to feel that you have lived your life, then it is meant to be pursued. If a dream seems happy without being acted upon, if it feels good to be left as a wish, then you may be content to leave it be.

Your dreams may be fueled or aligned with your passions, but they may not be the same thing. For example, you may be passionate about cooking, yet you may or may not dream of opening a restaurant. Instead, you may dream of taking a cooking class in France. Your greatest passions may lie in the realm of the outdoors, fueling a love of gardening and hiking, yet your greatest dream may have nothing to do with the outdoors; perhaps you dream of volunteering with disadvantaged children after retirement. Or perhaps your greatest passion does align with your dreams. You might be passionate about women's rights and dream of heading up a woman's advocacy center in your community.

Our passions often give us the fiery interest, motivation, and energy to accomplish our dreams. As we age, we often begin to give well-deserved attention to such seemingly minute, yet vital aspects of life. Perhaps this occurs as a gift of self-reflection, one that increasingly begins to honor the stalwart passage of time.

You might find yourself thinking, "I must follow my dreams, for if not now, when?" You might also be saying, "I'm too old to pursue my dreams. It's simply too late." I would say to you, "It's never too late to follow your dreams. You can pursue the life of your dreams until your last breath. Now is your time to begin."

Wisdom Tip 79: Pause to Imagine Your Dreams.

Pause to imagine your dreams. Dig into the crevices of your memory. Peer into the corners of your mind. Bring your dreams into focus. When you are ready, make a list of your dreams. Place no limits on your dreams; none are too silly, too wild, too small, or too big. Allow them to unfold without judgment on the page before you. Some may intersect with your passions and some may not.

Wisdom Tip 80: Attend to Your Dreams and Notice Your Wishes.

As you gaze at your list of dreams, allow yourself time to soak in their meaning and essence. Discern which are "wishes" (those that are content to live on as imaginings) and which are "musts" (those that beckon to you to be fulfilled). As with your passions, these "musts" are the dreams that are asking for your thoughtful attention. It is these dreams that crave to be part of your joyful journey into aging.

Wisdom Tip 81: Visualize Your Dreams Unfolding.

Smile. Imagine your dreams coming to life before your eyes. Imagine doing what must be done to make your dreams come true. Perhaps it's time to make a focused plan. Maybe it's time to set a few well-defined goals. It could be time to put yourself first and infuse your dreams with time, energy, and the necessary resources.

If the dreams before you feel undoable or difficult, remember to revisit "Nine Steps for Empowered Change" in chapter 2.

Wisdom Tip 82: Activate Your Dreams with Courage.

When you begin to take your dreams seriously, magic tends to happen. As you talk about your dreams and make them known to others, the little pieces often begin to come together. When you have the courage to share your dreams, positive energy is activated. As you start to act on your dreams, you are encouraging and supporting your process.

Wisdom Tip 83: Invite Others to Share in Your Dreams.

Invite others to share in your dreams. Sometimes a dream is truly meant to be shared with others. There are times that a dream wants to be shared privately with a friend or two, or maybe it wants to be enlivened with the support of one's family, friends, or community. And, sometimes, by sharing our dreams, we give others the opportunity to make their own dreams come true. Dreams put into action have a wonderfully infectious quality to them.

Many people have grand dreams for their lives. Some want to achieve notability in minor or magnificent ways. Some want to acquire power, mountains of material things, and extraordinary amounts of money. Some seek internal wealth and inner peace.

Others just want to get by, to get through life as unscathed and as safe as possible. We all might have big and little dreams somewhere along these various spectrums, with some dreams being externally focused and others directed toward the internal world. Every dream you have matters. Whether yours are large or small, each dream has a life—a potential—begging to be brought to the forefront. Whether your biggest goal in life is to put your child through college, own a home, create a successful business, or take a trip across the country, your dreams are your own. Please never devalue your dreams; do not compare them to the dreams of others. Your dreams are yours to be lived, now more than ever.

Our "must-do" dreams are vital to our lives. Yet I've found that it's not the dream that matters most, but the way we approach our own dreams in concert with the reality that life presents to us. It is the nature of this dance—our ability to weave our dreams with the reality of life—that ultimately seems to define our lives. You may wish to ask yourself these questions: When life brings me challenges, how do I respond? When an outcome isn't what I had hoped for or expected, what attitude do I take? When my dreams don't seem to be coming true, what do I do and what attitude do I take? Have I learned (or I am learning) to find the opportunities within life's vicissitudes?

Wisdom Tip 84: Explore How You Respond to Life's Challenges.

Once again, pause to ponder the question—*When life brings me challenges, how do I respond?* With this question in mind, consider a recent life challenge. Think about how you responded. In a nonjudgmental way, notice if there is any room for improvement for the future by looking at these three areas:

1. Can you reframe the situation to find a positive learning lesson?
2. Can you envision a way to embrace the challenge rather than fight it?

3. If you could redo this challenge, would you do anything differently?

If you can create a shift in any or all of these areas, notice that you have created a most powerful potential for change. All you need do is take this piece of learning and apply it to the next challenge that comes your way. It is not our challenges, but the way in which we respond to them, that makes the difference in our lives and the lives of others.

Wisdom Tip 85: Notice How You Respond to Disappointment.

Now focus on the question—*When an outcome isn't what I had hoped for or expected, what attitude do I take?* Envision a recent disappointment or challenge that had a less-than-hoped-for outcome. Notice if your attitude made the outcome harder to accept or more difficult in some other way. In a nonjudgmental way, consider if a shift in attitude would be helpful in the future. Consider if you can create a positive shift in these three areas:

1. Can you adjust your expectations to reduce your disappointment?
2. Can you envision a way to embrace the outcome rather than suffer from it?
3. If you could revisit the situation, would you do anything differently?

If you can create a shift in any or all of these areas, notice that your awareness is a powerful agent for change. When you apply this awareness to future situations, you will feel more accepting and positive about the outcome. An attitude of compassion for yourself and others will work magic.

Wisdom Tip 86: Appreciate Your Amazing Resilience.

You are an amazing woman who has been through so much in life. Pause in this moment to write a paragraph or more to honor your resilience; it is your resilience that has brought you thus far in your journey. Resilience is not a given in life; it is learned, earned, and fostered. Your resilience has allowed you to bend and not break during this journey of life. This beautiful resilience you have fostered will be your friend through every challenge that comes your way.

Wisdom Tip 87: Write a Letter of Gratitude to Your Wonderfully Courageous Self.

Indeed, you are a most courageous woman. Every segment of your life has asked you to dip into your inner courage in one way or another. Whether having the courage to foster a romantic relationship, have children, raise children, work within the home, work outside the home, make it through health challenges, face death, embrace loss, or simply thrive through the daily rigors of life, it is your courage that has allowed you to wake up to face each day. It is your courage that has allowed you to strive to be your best self one step at a time.

Pause to write a heartfelt letter of gratitude to the courageous woman that is you. Thank her. Honor her. Love her. Give her the gift of a loving letter to allow her to know that *you see her.*

I'll share a short, personal tale that makes me smile while it also brings tears to my eyes. My parents never had easy lives, but they were good souls. They worked hard, and they loved as best as they knew how. They made mistakes, but their success far outweighed their stumbles. It was during their later years that I came to know and love them in ways I never had before. My strong-willed, mercurial father was a difficult man in many ways. It was one of my greatest dreams in life to feel loved and seen by him. I desperately yearned for a kind, gentle touch from him, and I prayed for his accepting approval of me as a woman and daughter.

As my father's health deteriorated, it was difficult to see this once-strong man reduced to living in pain and fear. Although pulled in many directions and often feeling as if I had "five thousand other more pressing things to do," I would visit him almost daily. Sometimes we chatted gently, yet often he was distracted, agitated, or in pain. One day, as if it were a most urgent matter, he requested that I paint a bench for him. It was an odd demand, for the wrought-iron piece was new with a natural-toned finish that didn't need additional decoration. Yet he insisted that I paint it in shades of green, gold, burgundy, and copper.

At first, I responded to his seemingly nonsensical request with a gentle, "Dad, it's new and doesn't need painting. Adding those colors will make it look rather odd. It's truly lovely as it is."

He, ever so stubborn, resisted with his customary insistence, "It's what I want. Do what I ask. Would you just buy paint and paint for me? Could you just do as I ask?"

Of course, it was much less a request than a command, so I listened to him as I always did. I purchased the paints and necessary supplies. Each time I visited, I would kneel near him in the living room (where the outdoor bench had been placed) and I would paint as "Danny Boy" played in the background.

Whenever I told him the project was finished, he'd shake his head and say, "No, it's not finished yet. It's far from done."

His eyes had long since failed him, yet he "knew" more paint was needed. And so, instead of resisting, I decided to paint with passion. I painted colors on top of colors. I purchased additional hues of amber, moss, and champagne gold. I painted for the child in him. I painted for the child in me. The bench took on a life of its own as the colors swirled and melded. It took me weeks of painting before he was satisfied, but that was the true joy of it. That bench allowed us to connect with each other through paint strokes, time spent together, and the realization that it was me—of all his ten children—that he asked to paint that ridiculous bench. He asked because he knew I would do it. He knew it would be a bit of a tussle, but that I would make time for him. He knew that he was fading, but that my love for him would bring me to his side. He knew his power over me, the power of love and devotion.

I also knew that my time with him was short. On some level, I recognized that I would treasure that odd bench-painting time as "my time" with a most precious man; it was my last opportunity to fulfill my dream of feeling loved and seen by my father. More importantly, it was my opportunity to love and see him as the man and father that he *so* wanted to be. That singular bench became a testament to love, joy, passion, connection, and dreams come true. That strange looking, love-filled bench taught me that I can—that *we* can—find our heart's desire within almost anything.

Wisdom Tip 88: Appreciate Those Who Have Guided You in Life.

It is vital that we honor our teachers in life. Our greatest teachers come in a wide variety of forms, whether they are our parents, teachers, coaches, relationships, spouses, children, co-workers, mentors, heroes, or friends. Sometimes we might not appreciate the gift of a teacher or relationship until we take a backward glance. But in pausing to honor those who have been our teachers, we come to better appreciate those people, as well as the gifts they have given to us.

This is your opportunity to write out a list of your teachers and the gifts they have bestowed upon you. From this place of gratitude and humility, your love and inner joy will grow.

Wisdom Tip 89: Strive to Be the Role Model You Wish You Had and Desire to Be.

You are a teacher and a mentor to so many. Every day of your life, you are modeling for others—women and men of all ages—how to be in the world. Envision yourself as the teacher and mentor you want to be. Go out every day and do the best you can to be the role model that you wish you had. Go out each day and strive to be the mentor you want to be.

Wisdom Tip 90: Breathe into Today with Deep Joy.

Life may not bring you exactly what you want, but you can give your life exactly what you wish to give. Vow, every day, to give to your life the love, energy, and passion it deserves. Don't let your age define you. Don't let a mere number limit you. Today is your day. Make it count. Wake up each morning with one can-do vow and see it through. Then when you go to bed at night, pat yourself on the back for having lived one more joyful day.

A loving, joy-filled life is yours to embrace no matter what comes your way. The aging process—the living process—it not for the faint of heart. Perhaps your future holds the care of your ailing loved ones, be they parents or an aging partner. Perhaps your days will bring you the raising or care of grandchildren or continued responsibilities with your own children. Maybe you will find yourself working far past your retirement age. Your life might also bring you vast spaces of time and energy to volunteer. Perhaps your days will be long and leisurely. Perhaps they will be hectic and wild. Whatever they are, know that they are yours. Trust that you can find spaces within these days ahead to breathe into your passion. Let it come to life in all shapes and sizes. Let it rise and soar. For this is true: today—this very moment—is all that you have. We aren't promised a tomorrow, but we have all the promise of today to do with as we will. Today is your day to open new doors and fly off passionately into the world of your dreams.

I can't tell you what your future holds, but I can tell you that it holds great promise. I can affirm that whatever you want to create is within your power. You, with passion and perseverance, can manifest whatever you wish your life to be. This is no dull, colorless life that waits for you. This is no life that is dictated by the number of wrinkles on your face or the amount of gray in your hair. This is a canvas that is fresh and new, just waiting for you to paint, draw, write, and play.

And so, if life gives you a piece of paper and pen, then make poetry with all of your heart. If it doesn't give you what you need to create your poetry, then search for that paper, pen, or crayon until they're in hand. And if life gives you a seemingly strange opportunity to paint an odd bench or two, then paint with all your heart. Find the meaning in life's little moments. Find the joys and opportunities within the challenges. Embrace your passions and your dreams. And then breathe into your life—this very moment—as if it's all you have . . . for, indeed, it is.

Joyfully Living Your Dreams

*A*s we conclude this adventure together, I want to offer you one last story that illuminates a most courageous real-life journey. This beautiful story may touch a personal chord, for it reflects faith and bravery in action. Her journey may resonate deeply with you; it is filled with the pain, hope, determination, and rich personal blossoming of womanhood. Indeed, her tale is one that speaks to the truth that dreams can come true when we have faith and persevere. It is my hope that her tale reminds you that this same capacity is alive and well within you.

Let me introduce you to Louisa, a wonderful woman who came to me just as she turned sixty. After a thirty-plus-year relationship with a man to whom she'd been devoted, he unexpectedly chose to leave her for another woman. Though they had not been married, Louisa had considered theirs a lifelong commitment. Childless and alone, Lousia felt abandoned, for she had also lost her father and, more recently, her mother. When she came to me, Louisa was devastated and nearly immobilized by grief.

As we worked together, I came to appreciate so much about this woman. She was witty, resilient, sensitive, and strong. She was honest, devoted, and pure of heart. Yet with all of her goodness, she was suffering with anxiety, worrisome dreams, and somatic symptoms. Together, we labored to detangle the roots of her often-debilitating sadness and fears. Although tired and fragile, Louisa invested a great deal of time and effort in her psychological healing process. Indeed, the journey to my office was not a short one, yet Louisa made the two-hour trips diligently; she was intent on moving forward with her life. There were times when she felt hopeless, and I would tell her, "It's okay. I will hold hope for you. I've plenty of faith to share."

And so, this lovely woman continued on her journey with a spunky, if gentle, spirit. She explored her former relationship in the hope of understanding herself better. She addressed her significant financial fears with straightforward diligence. She allowed her few friends to support her, yet—as many of them were in need themselves—she found herself also supporting them. Surrounded by the cats who were her children, Louisa began to rebuild her life from the inside out.

During one appointment, Louisa asked if I thought she was ready for a new relationship. By this time, Louisa had been seeing me as needed for a little over one year. I smiled, looked into her sparkling eyes, and asked her if *she* felt ready for a new relationship.

She laughed quietly and said, "I think so, but I'm worried about it. I haven't dated in over thirty years. I wouldn't even know where to begin."

I smiled into her frightened eyes and said, "Ah, don't worry. You've great courage and strength, Louisa. Yes, it's a strange new world of dating out there, but you'll feel better about it once you've learned a few strategies."

So Louisa cautiously began to venture into the world of online dating. In a slow and hesitant way, sometimes feeling as if she'd taken one step forward and three steps back, Louisa began her journey into finding a new partner. There were times when things got a bit messy and confusing. Sometimes our sessions were spent addressing her dating-related frustrations and anxieties.

During one appointment, Louisa cried in frustration, noting, "I don't think I'm cut out for relationships. I think I am meant to be alone. I feel hopeless."

I empathized with her, for it was a difficult journey. "Don't worry, Louisa," I responded. "Even when you feel hopeless, I hold hope for you. I've plenty of hope to spare."

As always, Louisa would smile at my supportive affirmations; she, like all of us, wanted to feel seen, heard, and loved.

One day, a shaky, despairing Louisa arrived at my office with news. She'd been diagnosed with cancer—a particularly invasive form that left little chance for survival. Her physician had explained that the cancer would most likely take her life within six months or—if she were fortunate—a year. She was ready to give up; this news seemed impossible for her to bear. We spent our time together shoring up Louisa's psychological resources, and she left feeling encouraged enough to move forward. Nothing, not even cancer, was going to take this precious woman before her time.

As she moved forward with chemotherapy and every traditional treatment offered by her health providers, Louisa also thoroughly investigated alternative treatments. Although her energy and financial resources were deteriorating, Louisa engaged in an array of treatments that were most suited to her, and she made encouraging progress. As her weight dwindled and her much-treasured auburn hair fell out in clumps, Louisa persevered. Her inner light—the essence of her spirit—wavered now and again. Each time we met, no matter how hopeless she felt, I would remind her, "Louisa, I am holding hope for you. You can make it through this. I am here for you."

Month after month, Louisa maintained her course with fierce, if often fragile, inner strength. During the times when her energy was high, Louisa maintained an interest in finding a life partner, yet her health condition troubled her.

"Is it fair," she once asked, "for me to date when I have cancer? It's not right to try to bring another person into my life right now, is it?"

I smiled and responded, "Louisa, only you can decide if you really want to date at this time. If you've the energy, it may feel good for you to get out and connect with someone. Your responsibility rests in being honest with a prospective partner about your health. Indeed, there might be someone out there who would be honored to share your journey—the good and the difficult—with you."

Although delicate and often weary, Louisa engaged in dating once again. She found support in a woman's therapy group, her individual psychotherapy, and the self-care techniques she learned to utilize at home. Louisa found herself in a few situations that were not ideal, and she wisely, though sadly, moved on. There were times, indeed, when the combination of her health issues and the difficult world of dating left her feeling frustrated and despairing. As I placed a touch of healing oil on her during the end of these sessions, I would remind her, "Louisa, you are stronger than you know. Remember, I hold hope for your beautiful future, even when your own hope is fragile. Have faith."

Through her strength and the care of her doctors, Louisa's cancer moved into remission. There came a time in her journey several years later when a wonderful and worthy man moved into Louisa's life. Although his appearance and certain characteristics were far different from what Louisa had traditionally thought "right" for her, she gave him a chance given that he was a good and caring soul. Indeed, I sensed that Louisa had surely found the right fit when she told me he had begun going to chemotherapy with her and that he sat with her, rubbing her cold feet with his warm hands. Soon after, Louisa arrived to her appointment wearing her sweetheart's boots; in the most precious of ways, the boots on her feet seemed symbolic of their relationship—one that was grounded, solid, and serving both of them very well. A day came when I met her sweetheart; his eyes radiated with purity, love, and devotion. This wonderful man stayed by Louisa's side every step of the way and, together, they fought and conquered her cancer. Now many months later, the two are married and learning ever more about love.

As Louisa said recently, "I was beginning to think I would die single—a spinster left cold and alone. Although life has its new challenges—learning how to be married at my age isn't easy—I have the greatest joy of knowing companionship and love. And that has made all of what I've encountered through life worth it. I now know what it feels like to love deeply and be genuinely loved in return. I am so grateful. I am finally living the life I had secretly dreamed about for so long."

Louisa's story is most beautiful, for her journey has been one of incredible courage and strength. Life has never been easy for this dear soul, yet she has moved forward one step at a time. She was intent on finding the life of her dreams. Even when faced with one loss and challenge after the other, Louisa would not give up hope. And indeed, when her hope did falter, mine was there to lend loving support. For, in truth, that is our greatest gift in life—our ability and willingness to live in love and faith and to offer these gifts to others. As in many things, this is an area where women shine.

And so, trust that I support you and hold you in my heart as you move forward in your own journey. Know that I have faith and hope enough to share with you. When your light of faith feels dim, trust that hope and love are always there for you. When your light of faith feels strong, strive to share your light and love with others. You will find that your radiance grows the more you embrace your powers of love, faith, and joy. There is no time like now—these precious, mature years of life—to embrace a love-filled life. There is no better time than now to follow your joyful dreams.

Thank you, from the bottom of my heart, for taking this journey with me. It has been my joy, my privilege, and my deep delight.

With love and joy,
Carla Marie Manly, PhD

References

Chapter 1

1. Westerhof, Gerben J., Miche, Martina, Brothers, Allyson F., Barrett, Anne E., Diehl, Manfred, Montepare, Joann M., Wahl, Hans-Werner, Wurm, Susanne. *The influence of subjective aging on health and longevity: A meta-analysis of longitudinal data.* Psychology and Aging, Vol 29(4), Dec 2014, 793–802. Abstract retrieved August 19, 2018. http://psycnet.apa.org/doiLanding?doi=10.1037%2Fa0038016

2. Stephan, Yannick, Sutin, Angelina, and Terracciano, Antonio. "Subjective Age and Personality Development: A 10-Year Study." *Journal of Personality.* Volume 83, Issue 2. April 2015. Abstract retrieve August 19, 2018. https://onlinelibrary.wiley.com/doi/abs/10.1111/jopy.12090 (First published: 28 January 2014)

Chapter 2

1. Orth, Ulrich, Ero, R.Y., & Luciano, E. C.. Development of Self-Esteem from Age 4 to 94 Years: A Meta-Analysis of Longitudinal Studies. APA PsychNet. Retrieved 9/6/18 from: http://psycnet.apa.org/fulltext/2018-33338-001.html

2. Keyes, Corey L.M. and Westerhof, Gerben J. *Chronological and subjective age differences in flourishing mental health and major depressive episode.* Pages 67-74 | Received 18 May 2011, Accepted 31 May 2011, Published online: 25 Jul 2011. Abstract retrieved September 29, 2018. https://doi.org/10.1080/13607863.2011.596811

    https://www.tandfonline.com/doi/abs/10.1080/13607863.2011.596811

3. Lyubomirsky, Sonja, Sheldon, Kennon M., & Schkade, David. *Pursuing Happiness: The Architecture of Sustainable Change.* Review of General Psychology. 2005. Vol. 9., No. 2, 111-131. Retrieved 8/11/18:

    http://sonjalyubomirsky.com/wp-content/themes/sonjalyubomirsky/papers/LSS2005.pdf

4. The National Institute of Mental Health. Major Depression. Retrieved 2/17/18 from: https://www.nimh.nih.gov/health/statistics/major-depression.shtml

5. National Institute on Aging. NIH. *Depression and Older Adults.* Retrieved: 8/11/18 https://www.nia.nih.gov/health/depression-and-older-adults

6. The National Institute of Mental Health. "Any Anxiety Disorder." Retrieved 2/17/18 from www.nimh.nih.gov/health/statistics/any-anxiety-disorder.shtml

7. Anxiety and Depression Association of America: ADAA. "Facts & Statistics." Retrieved 1/30/18 from: https://adaa.org/about-adaa/press-room/facts-statistics#

8. Kwak, Seyul; Kim, Hairin, Chey, Jeanyung, and Youm, Yoosik. *Feeling How Old I Am: Subjective Age Is Associated with Estimated Brain Age.* Frontiers in Aging Neuroscience. 10: 168. Published online June 7, 2018. Article retrieved 9/29/18: https://www.ncbi.nlm.nih.gov/pmc/articles/PMC5999722/

Chapter 3

1. *Health screenings for women ages 40 to 64.* National Institutes of Health. U.S. National Library of Medicine. MedlinePlus. https://medlineplus.gov/ency/article/007467.htm

2. *Health screenings for women over age 65.* National Institutes of Health. U.S. National Library of Medicine. https://medlineplus.gov/ency/article/007463.htm

3. *The Physical Activity Guidelines for Americans.* JAMA Network. JAMA. November 20, 2018

    Katrina L. Piercy, PhD, RD1; Richard P. Troiano, PhD2; Rachel M. Ballard, MD, MPH3; et al. Retrieved December 16, 2018 from: https://jama-network.com/journals/jama/article-abstract/2712935

4. Exercise training increases size of hippocampus and improves memory. NCBI. Proc Natl Acad Sci U S A. 2011 Feb 15;108(7):3017-22. doi: 10.1073/pnas.1015950108. Epub 2011 Jan 31.

    Erickson KI1, Voss MW, Prakash RS, Basak C, Szabo A, Chaddock L, Kim JS, Heo S, Alves H, White SM, Wojcicki TR, Mailey E, Vieira VJ, Martin SA, Pence BD, Woods JA, McAuley E, Kramer AF. Retrieved 12/16/18: https://www.ncbi.nlm.nih.gov/pubmed/21282661

5. Cognitive Health and Older Adults. National Institute on Aging. (NIH). Retrieved 12/18/18 at: https://www.nia.nih.gov/health/cognitive-health-and-older-adults

6. Mechanisms of immunosenescence. Immunity and Aging: 2009; 6: 10. Published online 2009 Jul 22. doi: 10.1186/1742-4933-6-10. Calogero Caruso, Silvo Buffa, Giuseppina Candore, Giuseppina Colonna-Romano, Deborah Dunn-Walters, David Kipling, and Graham Pawelec. Retrieved 12/16/18: https://www.ncbi.nlm.nih.gov/pmc/articles/PMC2723084/

7. Duggal et al. Major features of Immunesenescence, including Thymic atrophy, are ameliorated by high levels of physical activity in adulthood. *Aging Cell,* 2018

Retrieved 12/1/18 from: https://www.ncbi.nlm.nih.gov/pubmed/29517845

8. *Properties of the vastus lateralis muscle in relation to age and physiological function in master cyclists aged 55–79 years.* Journal: Aging Cell Anatomical Society Authors: Ross D. Pollock, Katie A. O'Brien, Lorna J. Daniels, Kathrine B. Nielsen, Anthea Rowlerson, Niharika A. Duggal, Norman R. Lazarus, Janet M. Lord, Andrew Philp, Stephen D. R. Harridge. First published: 08 March 2018. https://doi.org/10.1111/acel.12735 Retrieved: 12/1/18: https://onlinelibrary.wiley.com/doi/full/10.1111/acel.127354

9. Cognitive Health and Older Adults. National Institute on Aging. (NIH). Retrieved 12/18/18 at: https://www.nia.nih.gov/health/cognitive-health-and-older-adults (This reference is the same as reference 5, above.)

10. The American Heart Association's Diet and Lifestyle Recommendations. Retrieved 12/18/18 from: https://www.heart.org/en/healthy-living/healthy-eating/eat-smart/nutrition-basics/aha-diet-and-lifestyle-recommendations

11. New Statistics Reveal the Shape of Plastic Surgery. American Society of Plastic Surgeons Report Shows Rise in Body Shaping and Non-Invasive Procedures. Press release Thursday, March 01, 2018. Retrieved 12/1/18 from: https://www.plasticsurgery.org/news/press-releases/new-statistics-reveal-the-shape-of-plastic-surgery

12. Ibid.

13. American Academy of Dermatology: Caring for Your Skin During Menopause. Retrieved 12/1/18: https://www.aad.org/public/skin-hair-nails/skin-care/skin-care-during-menopause

14. Aging and Painful Skin. Cleveland Clinic. Retrieved 12/1/18 at: https://my.clevelandclinic.org/health/diseases/16725-aging--painful-skin

15. CDC. Vaccines and Preventable Diseases What You Should Know About Zostavax. Retrieved 12/1/17 at: https://www.cdc.gov/vaccines/vpd/shingles/public/zostavax/index.html

16. Cleveland Clinic. Menopause, Perimenopause, and Postmenopause. Retrieved 12/1/18 from: https://my.clevelandclinic.org/health/diseases/15224-menopause-perimenopause-and-postmenopause

17. Mayo Clinic. Perimenopause. Retrieved 12/1/18 from: https://www.mayoclinic.org/diseases-conditions/perimenopause/symptoms-causes/syc-20354666

18. Mayo Clinic. Menopause. Retrieved 12/1/18 from: https://www.mayoclinic.org/diseases-conditions/menopause/symptoms-causes/syc-20353397

19. Mayo Clinic. Hot Flashes. Retrieved 12/1/18 from: https://www.mayoclinic.org/diseases-conditions/hot-flashes/symptoms-causes/syc-20352790

20. John Hopkins Medicine Health Library. Introduction to Menopause. Retrieved 12/14/18: https://www.hopkinsmedicine.org/healthlibrary/conditions/gynecological_health/introduction_to_menopause_85,P01535

21. National Institute of Health. U.S. Library of Medicine. Medline Plus. Hormone Replacement Therapy: Retrieved 12/1/18 from: https://medlineplus.gov/hormonereplacementtherapy.html

22. Dangor, Joe. News Network. Mayo Clinic. Mayo Clinic Newsroom. Oxybutynin lessens hot flash frequency, improves breast cancer survivor quality of life, Mayo-led study finds. Released December7, 2018. Retrieved 12/14/18: https://newsnetwork.mayoclinic.org/discussion/oxybutynin-lessens-hot-flash-frequency-improves-breast-cancer-survivor-quality-of-life-mayo-led-study-finds/

23. NCBI. National Institute of Health. Geller, Stacie and Studee, Laura. Botanical and dietary supplements for menopausal symptoms: What does and does not work. Retrieved 12/10/18: https://www.ncbi.nlm.nih.gov/pmc/articles/PMC1764641/

24. Centers for Disease Control. (Last updated March 29, 2018). Alcohol and public health: Frequently asked questions. Retrieved January 15, 2018, from https://www. cdc.gov/alcohol/faqs.htm.

   Wood, A. M., Kaptoge, S., Butterworth, A. S., Willeit, P., Warnakula, S., Bolton, T., Paige, E., et al. (April 14, 2018). Risk thresholds for alcohol consumption: combined analysis of individual-participant data for 599,912 current drinkers in 83 prospective studies. *The Lancet, 391*(1012), 1513–23. https://www.thelancet.com/journals/lancet/article/PIIS0140-6736(18)30134-X/fulltext.

25. NCBI. National Institute of Health. Effects of a dietary intervention and weight change on vasomotor symptoms in the Women's Health Initiative. Retrieved 12/10/18: https://www.ncbi.nlm.nih.gov/pmc/articles/PMC3428489/

26. Magkos, Faidon, Fraterrigo, Gemma, Yoshino, Jun, Okunade, Adewole, Patterson, Bruce, and Klein, Samuel. Cell Metabolism. Effects of moderate and subsequent progressive weight loss on metabolic function and adipose tissue biology in humans with obesity. Published February 22, 2016. DOI: https://doi.org/10.1016/j.cmet.2016.02.005. Retrieved 11/30/18 from: https://www.cell.com/cell-metabolism/fulltext/S1550-4131(16)30053-5?_returnURL=https%3A%2F%2Flinkinghub.elsevier.com%2Fretrieve%2Fpii%2FS1550413116300535%3Fshowall%3Dtrue

27. Villaverde-Gutiérrez C, Araújo E, Cruz F, Roa JM, Barbosa W, Ruíz-Villaverde G. Quality of life of rural menopausal women in response to a customized exercise programme. Journal of Advanced Nursing. 2006 Apr;54(1):11-9. Retrieved 12/3/18 from: https://onlinelibrary.wiley.com/doi/abs/10.1111/j.1365-2648.2006.03784.x

28. National Heart, Lung, and Blood Institute (NHLBI). (n.d.). Sleep deprivation and deficiency: Why is sleep important? Retrieved February 24, 2018, from https:// www.nhlbi.nih.gov/node/4605. Centers for Disease Control, 1 in 3 adults don't get enough sleep.

29. National Poll on Healthy Aging. University of Michigan. Urinary Incontinence: An inevitable part of aging? Retrieved 12/3/18 from: https://www.healthyaging-poll.org/sites/default/files/2018-10/NPHA_Incontinence-Report_FINAL-102318.pdf

30. Swan, Study of Women's Health Across the Nation. Retrieved 12/3/18 from: https://www.swanstudy.org/urinary-incontinence-problematic-for-many-wom-en-over-40-study-finds/ (Note: Original article by Sammy Caiola, Sacramento Bee 04/16/15.)

31. Urology Care Foundation. The American Urological Association. What is Overactive Bladder. Retrieved 12/3/18 from: http://www.urologyhealth.org/urologic-conditions/overactive-bladder-(oab)

32. Stewart WF, Van Rooyen JB, Cundiff GW, Abrams P, Herzog AR, Corey R, Hunt TL, Wein AJ. Prevalence and burden of overactive bladder in the United States. World Journal of Urology. 2003 May;20(6):327-36. Epub 2002 Nov 15. Abstract retrieved 12/3/18 from: https://www.ncbi.nlm.nih.gov/pubmed/12811491

33. US Department of Health and Human Services. Office on Women's Health. A Fact Sheet from the Office of Women's Health. Urinary Incontinence. PDF retrieved 12/3/18 from: https://www.womenshealth.gov/a-z-topics/urinary-incontinence

34. Danforth, Kim; Townsend, Mary; Lifford; Karen; Curhan, Gary; Resnick, Neil; Grodstein, Francine. Risk factors for urinary incontinence among middle-aged women. American Journal of Obstetrics and Gynecology. Volume 194, Issue 2, February 2006. Pages 339-345. Abstract retrieved 12/3/18 from: https://www.sciencedirect.com/science/article/pii/S000293780501135X

35. The National Association for Continence. Common Bladder Irritants. Retrieved 12/3/18 from: https://www.nafc.org/diet-and-exercise/

36. Cleveland Clinic. Menopause and Bladder Control. Retrieved 12/3/18 at: https://my.clevelandclinic.org/health/diseases/10081-menopause--bladder-control

37. University of Michigan. National Poll on Healthy Aging. Let's Talk About Sex. Retrieved 11/30/18: https://www.healthyagingpoll.org/report/lets-talk-about-sex

38. Twenge, Jean M.; Ryne A. Sherman, Ryne, A.; Wells, Brooke E. Declines in Sexual Frequency among American Adults, 1989–2014. Archives of Sexual Behavior. November 2017, Volume 46, Issue 8, pp 2389–2401. Full

article retrieved 12/3/18 from: https://link.springer.com/article/10.1007/s10508-017-0953-1

39. Graham, C., Mercer, C., Tanton, C., Jones, K., Johnson, A., Wellings, K., and Mitchell, K. What factors are associated with reporting lacking interest in sex and how do these vary by gender? Findings from the third British national survey of sexual attitudes and lifestyles. Full article retrieved 11/30/18 from: https://bmjopen.bmj.com/content/7/9/e016942#T2

40. Muise, A., Schimmack, U., and Impett, E. Sexual frequency predicts greater well-being, but more is not always better. Sage Journals. First published 11/18/15. https://doi.org/10.1177/1948550615616462 Abstract retrieved 11/30/18 from: https://journals.sagepub.com/doi/abs/10.1177/1948550615616462

41. Trompeter, S., Bettencourt, R., Barrett-Conner, E. Sexual Activity and Satisfaction in Healthy Community-dwelling Older Women. The American Journal of Medicine. January 2012Volume 125, Issue 1, Pages 37–43.e1. Abstract retrieved 11/30/18 from: https://www.amjmed.com/article/S0002-9343(11)00655-3/abstract

42. Lippe Taylor. Healthy Women. Women's Health Behavior Index. PDF retrieved 12/1/18 from: https://www.healthywomen.org/sites/default/files/LT_HW_Survey_1_Infographic_5.11.15.pdf

43. The Happiness Index: Love and relationships in America. eHarmony. Retrieved 12/1/18 from: https://www.eharmonyhappinessindex.com/

44. Office on Women's Health. U.S. Department of Health & Human Services: Menopause and sexuality. Retrieved 12/3/18 from: https://www.womenshealth.gov/menopause/menopause-and-sexuality

45. CDC. Centers for Disease Control & Prevention. Human papillomavirus: HPV. Retrieved 12/1/18 from: https://www.cdc.gov/hpv/parents/vaccine.html

46. CDC. Centers for Disease Control & Prevention. Retrieved 11/301/18 from: https://www.cdc.gov/std/general/default.htm

47. Mayo Clinic. Dementia. https://www.mayoclinic.org/diseases-conditions/dementia/symptoms-causes/syc-20352013

ACKNOWLEDGMENTS

It is a privilege and joy to honor those who have offered their love, support, and guidance throughout my life and the writing of this book.

Thank you, my dear parents, for your love and guidance; thank you for believing in me and always wanting me to be my best self.

Brian, our journey is one of teaching and learning in love; thank you for being in my life.

Adam, you are a brilliant treasure of love and light; thank you for all that you do and all that you are.

Cody, you are a precious beacon of power; thank you for your precious love.

Marisha, your time and energy have been most appreciated; your thoughtful, wise insights have been invaluable. Thank you for your generosity of wisdom and spirit. Your kindness, power, and light are inspiring for women of all ages.

Cali, I am most grateful for your kindness, positivity, and supportive presence in my life.

Linnea, thank you for your sweet, loving kindness and support.

Genevieve and Rich, you are my treasured adopted family; thank you for your loving friendship.

Jasmine, your loving friendship has made a vast difference in my life; thank you for your tremendous support.

Martell, your kind, loving feedback has been so appreciated; thank you for your caring generosity.

Erika, your friendship and love have made my life journey ever so sweet; thank you for your loving guidance.

Orchid, you are a most cherished friend and sister; thank you for your love and support.

Elise, your friendship and constancy are most precious to me.

Thomas Moore, you are a brilliant light of love and wisdom in my life; thank you for your friendship.

Laurie Duersch, the editing process was a joy because of you. Your kindness, diligence, and professionalism have allowed this book to shine. Thank you for lovely insights, guidance, and support.

Kate Farrell, your positive, enthusiastic marketing and PR efforts continue to amaze me; thank you for your dedication and support.

Brooke Jorden, your expertise and guidance have been most wonderful; thank you for your kindness.

Familius publishing team, thank you for your wonderful support and guidance.

I am blessed by every friend who has loved me, every mentor who has guided me, every teaching that has informed me, and every client who has reached out to me along the way. My life would not be what it is without you.

I am deeply grateful to you, the reader. Without your desire and willingness to learn and grow, I would not be able to share the passions that live within my mind, heart, and soul.

About the Author

Dr. Carla Marie Manly is a practicing clinical psychologist in Sonoma County, California. With her doctorate in clinical psychology and her master's degree in counseling, Dr. Manly merges her psychotherapy skills with her writing expertise to offer clear, insightful guidance. As an author, advocate, and speaker, she is tremendously passionate about helping others optimize their overall health and wellness. Whether working with individuals or groups, Dr. Manly's holistic, body-mind-spirit approach to psychotherapy focuses on creating love and healing from the inside out.

As a devoted wife, mother, and friend, Dr. Manly enjoys spending time with those she loves. Whenever possible, she enjoys practicing yoga, meditating, reading, walking, gardening, and baking. A passionate protector of nature, animals, and the less fortunate, she finds great joy in volunteering and taking positive action in life. Dr. Manly is an avid traveler and lover of the ocean, and she enjoys adventures that offer a blend of the beauty and wonder of life.

About Familius

Visit Our Website: www.familius.com

Familius is a global-trade publishing company that publishes books and other content to help families be happy. We believe that the family is the fundamental unit of society and that happy families are the foundation of a happy life. We recognize that every family looks different, and we passionately believe in helping all families find greater joy. To that end, we publish books for children and adults that invite families to live the Familius Nine Habits of Happy Family Life: *love together, play together, learn together, work together, talk together, heal together, read together, eat together,* and *laugh together.* Founded in 2012, Familius is located in Sanger, California.

Join Our Family

There are lots of ways to connect with us! Subscribe to our newsletters at www.familius.com to receive uplifting daily inspiration, essays from our Pater Familius, a free ebook every month, and the first word on special discounts and Familius news.

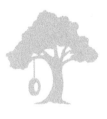

Connect

Facebook: www.facebook.com/paterfamilius
Twitter: @familiustalk, @paterfamilius1
Pinterest: www.pinterest.com/familius
Instagram: @familiustalk

The most important work you ever do will be within the walls of your own home.

CPSIA information can be obtained
at www.ICGtesting.com
Printed in the USA
FSHW022137310719